Trigger Point Therapy

for

Knee, Leg, Ankle, and Foot Pain

Valerie DeLaune, LAc

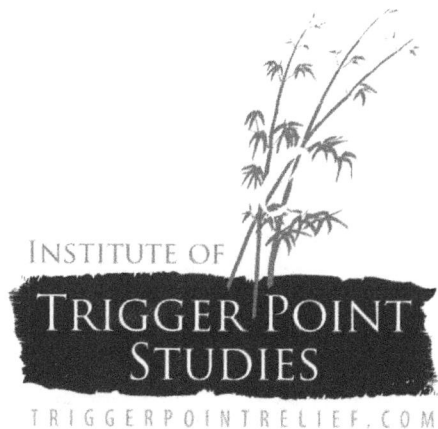

INSTITUTE OF
**TRIGGER POINT
STUDIES**
TRIGGERPOINTRELIEF.COM

ISBN 13: 978-0-9968553-4-1

First Edition, 2018

Disclaimer:

The following information is intended for general information purposes only. Individuals should always see their health care provider before administering any suggestions made in this book. Any application of the material set forth in the following pages is at the reader's discretion and is his or her sole responsibility.

This book is intended as a quick-reference only for the major muscles that may harbor trigger points that refer pain to the knee, leg, ankle, and foot areas. It is not intended as a comprehensive therapy guide for other areas of the body. If you are unable to relieve all of your pain with the techniques found in this book, you may wish to consult one of the resources found at the end of this book in order to treat other pertinent muscles.

Table of Contents

Acknowledgements / About the Author 1

Chapter 1: Knee, Leg, Ankle, and Foot Pain 3

Chapter 2: Locating and Treating Trigger Points: General Guidelines 14

Chapter 3: Trigger Point Location Guide 20

Chapter 4: Gluteus Minimus 24

Chapter 5: Quadriceps Femoris Muscle Group 31

Chapter 6: Adductor Muscles of the Hip 40

Chapter 7: Sartorius 44

Chapter 8: Hamstrings 47

Chapter 9: Popliteus 52

Chapter 10: Gastrocnemius 55

Chapter 11: Soleus / Plantaris 60

Chapter 12: Tibialis Posterior 65

Chapter 13: Peroneal Muscle Group 67

Chapter 14: Tibialis Anterior 71

Chapter 15: Long Flexor Muscles of the Toes 75

Chapter 16: Long Extensor Muscles of the Toes 78

Chapter 17: Superficial Intrinsic Foot Muscles 82

Chapter 18: Deep Intrinsic Foot Muscles 87

Appendix A: Perpetuating Factors 91

Appendix B: What Are Trigger Points? 111

Other Books by The Author 117

Acknowledgements

This book would not have been possible without the lifeworks of Dr. Janet Travell and Dr. David G. Simons, who worked endlessly to research trigger points, document referral patterns and other symptoms, and bring all of that information to medical practitioners and the general public. Together Doctors Travell and Simons produced a comprehensive two-volume text on the causes and treatment of trigger points, written for physicians. This text is a condensation of those volumes, written for the general public, and for practitioners who don't need the in-depth knowledge to perform trigger point injections.

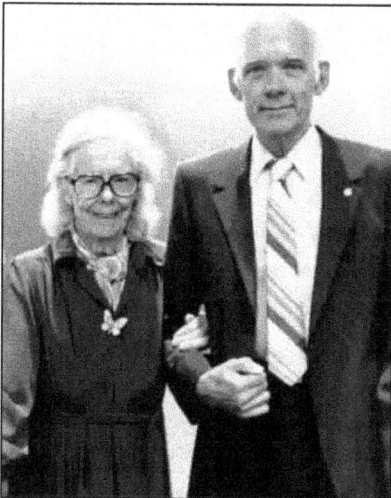

Dr. Janet Travell and Dr. David G. Simons

Dr. Travell pioneered and researched new pain treatments, including trigger point injections. In her private practice, she began treating Senator John F. Kennedy, who at the time was using crutches due to crippling back pain and was almost unable to walk down just a few stairs. It had become important for presidential candidates to appear physically fit, because of television. Being on crutches probably would have cost President Kennedy the election. Dr. Travell became the first female White House physician, and after President Kennedy died, she stayed on to treat President Johnson. She resigned a year and a half later to return to her passions: teaching, lecturing, and writing about chronic myofascial pain. She continued to work into her nineties and died at the age of ninety-five on August 1, 1997.

Dr. Simons met Dr. Travell when she lectured at the School of Aerospace Medicine at Brooks Air Force Base in Texas in the 1960s. He soon teamed up with Dr. Travell and began researching the international literature for any references to the treatment of pain. There were a few others out there who were also discovering trigger points but using different terminology. He studied and documented the physiology of trigger points in both laboratory and clinical settings and tried to find scientific explanations for trigger points. He continued to research the physiology of trigger points, update the trigger point volumes he coauthored with Dr. Travell, and review trigger point research articles until his death at the age of 88 on April 5, 2010.

I am also profoundly grateful to my neuromuscular therapy instructor, Jeanne Aland, who taught me basics about trigger points, and introduced me to the books written by Doctors Travell and Simons. I was told Jeanne passed on a few years ago.

All three are well-missed. Those familiar with trigger points are extremely grateful for their hard work and dedication. Their work lives on through the hundreds of thousands of patients who have gotten relief because of their research and willingness to train others.

Other Thanks

Many additional researchers have contributed to the study of trigger points, and many doctors and other practitioners have taken the time to learn about trigger points and give that information to their patients. I would like to acknowledge all of them for their role in alleviating pain by making this important information available. In particular I would like to thank Dr. Juhani Partanen, who kindly explained the "Muscle Spindle" hypothesis to me in lay terms, and also took the time to review the chapter "Appendix B: What Are Trigger Points?" to make sure I had translated scientific language correctly into easier-to-understand terms.

My Background

I attended massage school in 1989 and learned Swedish massage. I learned to give a very good general massage, but I didn't feel equipped to treat chronic pain. I was very intrigued by a description of a continuing education certificate course; it was called *neuromuscular therapy*, which combines *myofascial release* (a type of deep tissue massage) with treating trigger points. I attended the class in 1991, taught by Jeanne Aland at Heartwood Institute, and it completely changed my approach to treating patients. Once I learned about referral patterns, I was able to consistently resolve chronic pain problems.

Over my years of treating thousands of patients, I have added my own observations to those of Doctors Travell and Simons, and developed a variety of self-help techniques, which are included in my books.

In 1999, I received my master's degree in acupuncture. Since then I've been writing trigger point books and articles, teaching trigger point continuing education classes to health care providers, and specializing in treating pain syndromes by combining dry-needling of trigger points with Traditional Chinese Medicine diagnosis and treatment.

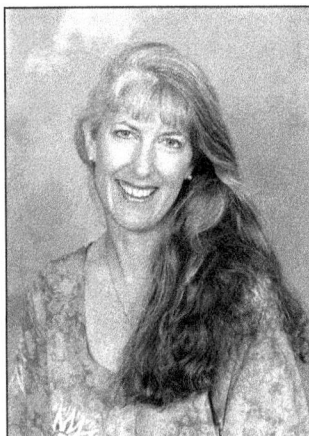

Valerie DeLaune, LAc

Chapter 1: Knee, Leg, Ankle, and Foot Pain

Incidences of leg and foot pain are on a dramatic rise due to an increase in the number of acute injuries, and because of the increasing number of people with medical conditions that affect the legs. The associated medical costs are staggering.

Acute injuries are most often due to sports injuries caused by improper training (including "weekend warrior" syndrome). If you are a sports enthusiast, properly warming up with stretches and mild exercise will go a long way toward preventing injuries. "Cross-training," or exercises that use different muscle groups in different ways, help by strengthening multiple muscle groups. If you only participate in one or two sports, you will only strengthen certain muscles, allowing others to be deconditioned. This sets you up for acute and chronic injuries, and leads to the formation of trigger points.

Chronic medical conditions such as diabetes, atherosclerosis, and obesity, which are most often the result of a sedentary lifestyle combined with a poor diet, can also indirectly cause and perpetuate trigger points. Because the muscles in the legs and feet support the entire weight of the body, they can be particularly susceptible to mechanical stresses, and because they are farthest from the heart, they are more likely to suffer from the poor circulation characteristic of these medical conditions.

This chapter addresses the most common sources of pain from injuries and chronic conditions, and how trigger points can potentially be involved either directly or indirectly.

Knee Pain

There can be several causes of knee pain, such as osteoarthritis, problems with the kneecap alignment, inflammation of one of the lubricating sacs of fluid in the knee (true bursitis), and damage to the cartilage, tendons, and ligaments either from overuse injuries or sudden traumatic injuries. If you had a sudden impact to your knee or leg and are experiencing severe pain in the knee area, you will want to see a doctor to be evaluated for structural damage.

If you have been diagnosed with some kind of tear or rupture, surgery may be necessary to repair the damage. Trigger point self-help techniques will be valuable pre- and post-surgery to keep the muscles as relaxed as possible, to speed healing, and to help minimize the potential long-term effects of peripheral and central sensitization.

Pain that has come on gradually is more likely due to an overuse injury or an inflammatory process such as bursitis or a degenerative condition such as osteoarthritis. Try the trigger point self-help techniques included in this book to see if you can relieve pain. If you can't reduce or relieve your pain fairly quickly, you will want to see a health care provider for an evaluation for structural damage. No matter what the cause, you will want to continue to apply pressure to trigger points.

Some of the more common problems affecting the knee are worth mentioning in more detail, especially those that can either be caused by or cause trigger points, such as osteoarthritis, patellofemoral pain, iliotibial band syndrome, tendinopathies and muscle strains, bursitis, meniscus tears, and ligament sprains and tears.

Osteoarthritis

Osteoarthritis (OA) is the most common joint disorder, and the knee is the joint most commonly affected. The cartilage cushioning the knee joint wears away first and then, as the degeneration progresses, the underlying bone can also wear away. This degeneration process causes the ends of the bones to become thicker, and they may form *osteophytes,* or spurs. It is presently unclear at which stage in the degeneration process that the joint becomes painful. While pain from OA is usually localized to the affected joint, hip OA may cause knee pain.

Symptoms may include a deep aching pain in the joint that gets worse after exercise or when putting weight on it, stiffness, limited mobility, a grating sound, joint swelling, and pain that is worse at night and with rainy weather. Resting the joint gives you relief. In the earlier stages, the pain may be episodic, but in advanced stages pain may be constant.

Risk factors are age, obesity, muscle weakness, and past injury. Women are affected more often than men. Almost half of American adults may develop osteoarthritis in at least one knee by age 85, with the likelihood increasing both with age, and as body mass increases with weight problems. Sixty-six percent of obese adults will develop osteoarthritis in one or both knees. Other risk factors include structural malalignment, muscle weakness, genetic predisposition, and certain professions that require hard labor, heavy lifting, knee bending, and repetitive motion. Once knee osteoarthritis degeneration starts, it becomes a vicious cycle. Your knee hurts, so you exercise less, which leads to muscle weakness and possibly to weight gain, which adds to the degeneration progression.

Both osteoarthritis and inflammatory joint disease can induce pain beyond the region of the joint and eventually form trigger points in the surrounding muscles. This may be why people with joint replacements still experience pain—it could be a result of trigger point pain referral, even though trigger points were not originally part of the underlying disease.

While advancing age and genetic predisposition are not within your control, modifying your work environment with correct ergonomic furniture and changing the way you use your body, along with changing your diet (if necessary) are things you can do fairly easily and relatively inexpensively. Structural malalignments and muscle weakness can be corrected with the help of a doctor, chiropractor, or physical therapist. You can do a lot to help stop the progression of osteoarthritis, or prevent it before it starts. Many of the self-help techniques in this book will be very helpful for treating trigger points that have already formed and preventing additional trigger points from forming.

Patellofemoral Pain (Chondromalacia Patellae)

The kneecap (patella) is a small bone with some cartilage on the side closest to the joint. The cartilage provides shock absorption and allows the kneecap to move smoothly through a groove that is formed by the ends of the leg and thigh bones (tibia and femur), located behind the kneecap. Pain around the kneecap that develops gradually is usually caused by muscle imbalances, where the *vastus lateralis* and *rectus femoris* muscles are tight, and the *vastus medialis* is not conditioned. This pulls the kneecap a little toward the outside of the leg, and it no longer tracks properly in the groove. The cartilage rubs against the underlying bone, and gets damaged over time. If the cartilage is damaged by an impact to the front of the kneecap, it can cause small tears or roughening of the cartilage, leading to pain.

If the cartilage has been damaged, symptoms may include a grinding or clicking when you are straightening your knee, pain that is worse when walking downstairs, pain upon standing up after sitting for a long period, possibly pain when pressing against the kneecap, and maybe slight swelling.

Muscle imbalances are usually easily solved by using the self-help techniques for trigger points found in the *vastus lateralis* and *rectus femoris* muscle chapter (5), and by strengthening the *vastus medialis* muscle. If the cartilage is not damaged, relief should be fairly quick. Other muscle groups that may benefit from treatment are the gluteal muscles and the *tensor fascia latae*, which are beyond the scope of this book. Correcting for foot pronation may also help, and is addressed in Appendix A.

If the cartilage has been damaged, surgery may be necessary, but as noted above, the techniques in this book will help you both pre- and post-surgery, and also help the realign the kneecap and prevent further damage.

Iliotibial Band Syndrome (Runner's Knee)

The iliotibial band (IT band) is connective tissue that attaches to the top of your pelvis and the tensor fascia latae muscle, runs down the side of the leg, and attaches on the outside of the tibia just below the knee. If the IT band is tight, as is common in runners, it can rub across the bony prominence at the bottom of the femur on the outside of the knee.

Symptoms may include pain on the outside of your knee that is worse with running, tightness along the outside of your thigh, pain when flexing and extending your lower leg, weakness in moving your leg out away from your body, and tightness in the gluteal and tensor fascia latae muscles.

True IT band syndrome can be confused with referred pain from trigger points in the posterior portion of the *gluteus minimus* (chapter 4), the *tensor fascia latae*, and *vastus lateralis* (chapter 5) muscles, since referred pain from trigger points in the first two muscles is felt on the outside of the thigh, and the *vastus lateralis* refers pain both over the outside of the thigh and into the knee. Because this book only addresses trigger points and referred pain from the knee on down and not the thigh, self-help techniques are only included for the *gluteus minimus* and *vastus lateralis* muscles. By working on these muscles, you can likely reduce or eliminate pain from IT band syndrome, but you may want to see the Resources section at the end of this book for books that cover additional muscles.

Quadriceps and Patellar Tendinopathy

The quadriceps tendon attaches your quadriceps muscle to your kneecap, and the patellar tendon runs from your kneecap to the tibia (the larger of the two lower leg bones). If stress is placed on the tendons, they can develop tiny tears (previously known as tendinitis or tendinosis). Tendons heal more slowly than muscles because they don't have as great a blood supply.

A variety of factors may be involved in developing tendinopathies, including sudden increases in the intensity and frequency of exercise, misalignment of your leg bones, muscular imbalances, tight thigh and other leg muscles, and being overweight. Symptoms may include an increase in pain and maybe a crunchy sound or feeling when using the tendon, and/or increased pain and stiffness at night or upon waking; the area may also be tender, red, warm, or swollen. The symptoms can easily be confused with bursitis. Treating trigger points using the methods taught in this book can relieve the tightness of muscles pulling on the tendons, prevent further damage to the tendons, reduce or stop pain, and allow the tendons to heal.

Hamstrings / Biceps Femoris Tendinopathy and Strains

Tightness in the hamstring muscles (chapter 8) can also stress and cause injuries to both the muscles and the associated tendons, for the same reasons as noted above for the quadriceps muscles. The hamstring tendons attach on the bones of the lower leg, just below the knee area.

Symptoms of tendinopathy include pain with pressure over the tendon attachment, pain with bending your knee combined with resistance pressure against the calf, and stiffness after exercise. Treating hamstring muscle trigger points using the methods taught in this book can relieve the tightness of muscles pulling on the tendons, prevent further damage to muscles and the tendons, reduce or stop pain, and allow the tendons to heal. If the biceps femoris tendon is completely torn (which is only likely with a rapid movement as required by certain sports), the torn area will swell. If you have swelling or severe pain, you will need to see a doctor for treatment and evaluation. Treating the tight muscles and trigger points can help prevent this kind of injury, as a relaxed muscle is less prone to injury than a tight one.

Bursitis

Though *true* bursitis may have little to do with trigger points except possibly indirectly (if the ligament or tendon from a tight muscle contributes to the friction that may be causing bursitis), I wanted to mention it because often pain in or over the joint is misdiagnosed as bursitis, when in fact it is actually referred pain from trigger points.

A *bursa* is a small fluid-filled sac that allows skin, tendons, muscles, and ligaments to slide easily over the underlying bone. Bursa sacs are found in and near joints such as the knee, over the trochanter of the femur bone (what most people would point to as their hip bone area), shoulder, and elbow. Bursitis of the knee can be caused by a traumatic blow to the bursa, by repeated pressure leading to irritation (such as repeated kneeling, as in the old terms "housemaid's knee" or "clergyman's knee"), and by infections. Symptoms include pain and tenderness on and just below the kneecap, pain with kneeling, and possibly swelling and warmth or even an abscess or fluid-filled lump. I believe it is worth checking for trigger points in the muscles surrounding the joint, just in case trigger points and tight muscles are causing the friction and irritating the bursa sac, or in case it is not really bursitis causing your knee pain.

Meniscus Tears

The lateral and medial menisci are cartilage that act as shock absorbers for the knee. Damage can be from an acute injury or degenerative changes, and damage to the medial meniscus is more common.

Symptoms may include swelling, tenderness or pain on the inside or outside of your knee located right next to the joint that is increased by bending your knee, and possibly audible sounds of popping, cracking, or clicking. This needs to be diagnosed by a doctor. If you had a sudden injury accompanied by a sound, you will certainly need to see a doctor for evaluation. If a tear is found, depending on the extent of the injury, the treatment may either be conservative—including icing, pain medications, ultrasound or laser therapy, massage/manual therapy, and eventually conditioning exercises—or surgery if the damage is more severe. Herbs and other supplements for healing traumatic injuries as well as acupuncture will be helpful. With either the conservative or surgical options, self-compression of trigger points will be helpful, as long as you don't stress your joints. Do not perform stretches without the guidance of your health care practitioner. Use pain as a guideline: if it hurts, don't do it—at least until you are under the supervision of a physical therapist.

Knee Ligament Sprains and Tears

Ligaments are connective tissue that attach bone to bone. In the knee, the two cruciate ligaments and the medial collateral ligaments attach the femur to the tibia. The lateral collateral ligament attaches the femur to the head of the fibula, the thinner bone in the lower legs.

Damage is usually caused by an injury as opposed to overuse, and can lead to or be found in combination with a meniscus tear (see above) or an injury to the articular cartilage (a pad between the femur and the tibia). Symptoms can range from mild tenderness over the ligament for a mild injury, to pain and knee instability if there is a complete tear of the ligament, and possibly swelling depending on which ligament is affected and the severity of the injury. The treatments under meniscus tears also apply to knee ligament tears.

Calf Pain

There are two large muscles in the calf—the *gastrocnemius* (chapter 10) and the *soleus* (chapter 11)—along with some other smaller muscles. Trigger points in these muscles can make them very susceptible to injury, and can also greatly impair your mobility.

If you have poor circulation in your legs due to conditions such as atherosclerosis or diabetes, you will be even more susceptible to developing trigger points in the legs and feet. The more severe the circulation impairment, the more trigger points, the more pain and reduced ability to exercise, leading to a worsening of the underlying disease.

Some of the more common conditions affecting the calves are muscle strains, compartment syndromes, periosteal stress (formerly shin splints), cramping, tendinopathies and tendon ruptures, and stress fractures. These can all be caused by trigger points that go undiagnosed and untreated.

Calf Muscle Strains

A muscle *strain* is damage to the muscle fibers, while a *sprain* refers to ligament damage. Strains are "graded" according to the amount of damage. A grade 1 strain is a minor tear, with up to 10 percent of the muscle fibers damaged. Symptoms may include a small amount of pain with tightness and aching for two to five days after the injury, and you can still tolerate using the muscles. A grade 2 strain is damage of up to 90 percent of the muscle fibers, and you will likely feel sharp pain that is worse with walking, along with tightness and aching of the affected area for a week or more, and there will be bruising and swelling. A grade 3 is a full rupture, with more than 90 percent torn muscle fibers. Pain will be severe and there will be a lot of bruising and swelling, and the muscle will bunch up near the top of the calf, which is often described as "a window blind rolling up suddenly."

Calf strains are usually caused by sudden forces being applied to tight calf muscles. You should consider a grade 1 or 2 injury as a warning sign to use the techniques found in this book before you suffer from a complete rupture and possibly require immediate surgery.

Compartment Syndromes

A *muscle compartment* is a group of muscles within a particular part of the body, wrapped by strong, fibrous tissue (fascia). The fascia attaches the compartment to the bone, and each compartment has a blood and nerve supply. For example, the lower leg contains four muscle compartments: The superficial posterior compartment contains the *soleus* and *gastrocnemius* muscles, and the deep posterior compartment contains the *flexor digitorum longus, flexor hallucis longus, popliteus,* and *posterior tibialis* muscles. The anterior compartment contains the *tibialis anterior, extensor hallucis longus, extensor digitorum longus,* and *peroneus tertius.* The lateral compartment contains the *peroneus longus* and *peroneus brevis* (see subsequent chapters on these muscles, and to see their locations).

A *compartment syndrome* is where increased pressure within the muscle compartment adversely affects blood and lymph circulation of the muscles inside. The most noticeable symptom is tightness, dull aching, and diffuse tenderness over the entire belly of the involved muscles. One or more of the muscles swell, causing pain and odd sensations, and the symptoms are worse with activity. Symptoms develop over time, and pain persists for increasing amounts of time after exercise. It is important to see a doctor *immediately.* If left untreated, compartment syndrome eventually causes scarring of the muscles and nerves and other permanent damage. A positive diagnosis is determined by measuring intramuscular pressure within the compartment. Once successfully treated by relieving pressure within the compartment, you should subsequently check for trigger points, since they were likely formed as a result of compartment syndrome.

Shin Splints and Tibial Periosteal Stress Syndromes

Anterior compartment syndrome is sometimes called "anterior shin splints," which is easily confused with the generic term "shin splints" used in the past to refer to any chronic pain in the front or middle of the lower leg associated with exercise. More recently, "shin splints" has come to refer specifically to irritation of the surface of the bone along the attachment of a muscle, and is called *periosteal irritation.* In the front of the leg, periosteal irritation may develop when a runner first changes from a flat-footed to a toe-running style, begins training on a track or hill (especially downhill), or runs in a shoe that is either too rigid or too flexible. Trigger point self-help techniques will help resolve periosteal irritation.

Calf Cramping

Calf cramps occurs most often when you are sleeping, or sitting for too long with your toes pointed. They are one of the most common symptoms of *gastrocnemius* (chapter 10) trigger points, though other calf muscles may be involved. Calf cramps may also be brought on by dehydration, loss of or inadequate intake of electrolytes (including potassium, calcium, magnesium, and salt), hypoparathyroidism, Parkinson's disease, and possibly diabetes.

If you are experiencing calf cramps, in addition to using the self-help techniques in subsequent chapters, try increasing your water intake and take a multimineral supplement. If you limit your salt intake severely or sweat heavily, try increasing your salt intake, unless otherwise directed by a doctor. Some drugs can cause calf cramps, such as lithium, cimetidine, bumetanide, vincristine, and phenothiazines. Taking vitamin E (400 IU per day) helps some people a great deal. If you take a multivitamin, be sure to count that amount of vitamin E toward the 400 IU, and only take the larger dose for a maximum of two weeks, or less if the cramps disappear more quickly. Try vitamin B_2 (riboflavin) if you have calf cramps during pregnancy.

Achilles Tendinopathy and Ruptures

The Achilles is the large tendon at the back of the ankle area that attaches the *gastrocnemius* (chapter 10) and *soleus* (chapter 11) muscles to the heel bone. This tendon enables you to flex and extend your foot, allowing you to walk or run.

As with the other tendinopathies mentioned above, Achilles tendinopathy is caused by micro trauma to the tendon rather than a long-term inflammatory process. Damage can occur over the course of a few days or over a longer period of time, depending on your activities.

Symptoms of acute Achilles tendinopathy may include pain at the beginning of an exercise that decreases as you continue to exercise, tenderness with pressure on the Achilles, and pain that decreases with rest. Symptoms of chronic tendinopathy may include pain that develops over a period of weeks or months, pain throughout exercise, pain that is worse when walking uphill or up stairs, pain and stiffness (particularly in the morning or after resting), tenderness with pressure on the tendon, nodules or lumps on the tendon, swelling or thickening over the tendon, and possibly redness on the skin. There is also a bursa sac on the back of the heel that can become irritated as part of Achilles tendinopathy, a condition called retrocalcaneal bursitis. Symptoms may include pain on the back of the heel (especially when running uphill or on soft surfaces), tenderness and swelling, and a spongy resistance when pressing on the area.

Causes of Achilles tendinopathy may include an increase in activity (distance, speed, or hills), change of footwear or your training surface, lack of adequate recovery time between activities, wearing heels (even low ones), foot pronation, weak calf muscles, and tight calf muscles that decrease range-of-motion at the ankle joint and stress the Achilles tendon. The self-help techniques found in subsequent chapters of this book will take the stress off the Achilles tendon and allow it to heal.

If the calf muscles are chronically tight, and you make abrupt movements, as with sports, you may get a partial or complete Achilles tendon rupture. Symptoms of a partial rupture may include a sudden, sharp pain in the Achilles tendon (or within twenty-four hours of the injury), sharp pains that come back at the beginning of exercise and then again after exercise has stopped, stiffness in the Achilles first thing in the morning, and slight swelling. A total rupture feels like someone has hit you hard on the calves with something, often accompanied by a loud sound. There will be a large amount of swelling, and you won't be able to walk well or stand on tiptoes. You may need to have surgery within two days in order for the injury to heal properly. Surgery has a lower re-rupture rate than nonsurgical options, but all surgeries have risks of complications. It is advisable to treat the calf muscles with self-help techniques before you rupture the tendon. If you have already ruptured the tendon, seek medical treatment and then perform the self-help techniques in this book to prevent re-injury.

Stress Fractures of the Tibia or Fibula

Symptoms of a stress fracture of the tibia (the larger of the two lower leg bones) may include pain that occurs after running long distances, tenderness and swelling over the site of the fracture (usually in the lower third of the lower leg), and pain when you press on the "shin bone." Stress fractures of the fibula are less common, and the pain will be located more over the outside of the lower leg rather than over the tibia.

Causes of tibial fractures include overloading the bones by long-distance running, a sudden change in running surface, and numerous cumulative small impacts to the bones. Causes of fibular fractures include tightness of the muscles surrounding the bone placing torque on the bone, and foot pronation. Using the techniques found in this book will help prevent fractures, and will also heal and prevent further injury if you have had a fracture.

Deep Vein Thrombosis

Deep vein thrombosis (DVT) is a blood clot in a vein, most common in the calf, which is most likely to occur after surgery or a long airplane ride. You are more at risk for DVT if you are over fifty, have poor circulation, or are overweight. It is potentially fatal if the clot works its way loose and travels to the heart, lung, or brain. Symptoms may include constant calf pain, swelling, heat in the area, deep tenderness in the muscle, and sometimes a localized reddening of the skin. If you think you are experiencing the symptoms of DVT, you should not receive massage of any kind, and you should seek medical help immediately for evaluation. Do NOT perform the techniques on the calf muscles found in this book, as pressure can help loosen the clot.

Ankle and Foot Pain

Your ankles and feet support the weight of your entire body. They are your foundation, shock absorber, balance mechanism, and means of getting around. One-quarter of the bones in the human body (twenty-six) are in the feet. There are thirty-three joints, and more than one hundred muscles, tendons, and ligaments. A problem that develops in the ankles and feet affects the entire body, such as when you limp or have to be on crutches while healing.

The most common problems affecting the ankles and feet are sprains, muscle and tendon tightness and subsequent damage, tibialis posterior syndrome, plantar fasciitis, stress fractures, hallux valgus, and toe drop.

Ankle Sprains

It is estimated that between twenty-three- and twenty-seven thousand lateral ankle sprains occur daily in the United States alone, though actual occurrences are probably significantly higher because as many as 55 percent of people with sprains may not seek treatment from a health care professional. Once an ankle has been sprained, the chance of spraining it again is greater than 70 percent, due to the injury to multiple structures in the ankle as well as changes in the central nervous system function that maintains a balance-feedback system, known as the "sensimotor system."

The most common ankle sprain is due to stretching or tearing of the lateral (outside) ligaments. It is possible to sprain the medial ligament (located on the "medial" side of the ankle, which is the side closest to the other ankle), but that occurs more often in conjunction with a fracture. Sprained ankles, as with all ligaments sprains, are divided into grades 1, 2, or 3, depending on their severity.

Mild sprains may only cause some discomfort. As the sprain increases in severity, you may also experience increasing amounts of swelling and bruising, pain, and joint instability. If your ankle is severely sprained, you may have ruptured ligaments and dislocated the ankle joint. There may also be damage to the tendons and other joint tissues, and small fractures, so you may need to get an X-ray to determine the extent of damage.

Foot pronation and supination may make you more susceptible to ankle sprains, so flat shoes with wide bases (no heels) are advisable, along with orthotics that stabilize your foot (see Appendix A). Calf muscles tighten up in response to an ankle sprain, so you will want to do the self-help techniques contained in subsequent chapters of this book to relieve tightness and prevent future injuries.

Peroneal Muscle and Tendon Damage

The *peroneus longus*, *brevis* and *tertius* are found along the outside of the lower leg. Symptoms of tendinopathy may include swelling on the outside of the ankle or heel, and pain that increases with activity, when pressing on the tendons, and when your foot is moved in certain directions. Causes include running on side-slanted surfaces (such as a road), overuse, foot pronation, and tight calf muscles, particularly the *peroneal* muscles. An ankle sprain can cause the peroneal tendons to slip forward over the outer ankle bone (lateral malleolus). A tight *peroneus brevis* muscle can cause a rupture of the tendon. Focus on the *peroneal* muscles (chapter 13) and see the section "Mechanical Stresses" in Appendix A. Self-help techniques will help prevent injuries.

Tibialis Posterior Syndrome

Tibialis posterior syndrome is another tendinopathy. The *tibialis posterior* is on the back of the leg, "deep to" the *gastrocnemius* and *soleus*, that is, it's the muscle right next to the lower leg bones. Pain will most likely be felt on the bottom of the foot, and there may be swelling around the middle ankle bone (medial malleolus). Foot pronation predisposes you to this injury, which is easily corrected with good orthotics and shoes with good heel bases. Do the self-help techniques found in chapter 12 to relax the *tibialis posterior* muscle belly, which will help relax the tendon.

Plantar Fasciitis, Heel Spurs, and Heel Pain

Heel pain can be caused by a number of conditions, including a bruised heel or even fractured heel (caused by repetitive pounding as in running), calcaneal bursitis, tarsal tunnel syndrome, plantar fasciitis, or referred pain from calf muscles, primarily the *soleus* (chapter 11). By far the most common sources of heel pain are the last two, and their relationship to each other. Unfortunately many practitioners aren't familiar with trigger points, so the true source of heel pain goes undiagnosed and untreated.

Plantar Fasciitis

Contrary to its name ("-itis") and what was originally thought, plantar fasciitis is not an inflammatory process, but rather is caused by tension overload on the plantar aponeurosis (the flat, broad tendons found between your heel and the ball of your foot) fascial attachment on the big bone in the heel. This tension overload is caused by tightness in the *gastrocnemius, soleus, abductor hallucis, flexor digitorum brevis,* and/or *abductor digiti minimi* muscles. The *quadratus plantae* may also be involved.

Pain from plantar fasciitis develops gradually, but will initially be more noticeable after an increase in athletic activity. Pain is worse in the morning, with your first steps being extremely painful until the muscles and plantar fascia have been stretched. Pain often is worse again in the evening, and after running or jumping. Foot pronation adds to the problem.

Treating trigger points, receiving ultrasound, and getting good orthotics with arch supports and deep heel cups are effective therapies. You will need to avoid running, jumping, and possibly walking until symptoms have decreased. You may need to lose weight, if necessary, since additional weight puts a lot of stress on the lower leg and foot structures. Numerous repeated injections of steroids can lead to rupture of the plantar aponeurosis, so you should use the above treatments first. The longer the condition goes on and the more you limp, the more muscles get involved, all the way up through the back and neck, so you should not wait to start treatment.

Heel Spurs

A heel spur is a little extra piece of bone that forms somewhere on the *calcaneus*, or heel bone, on the side closest to the ball of your foot. You may have heel spurs with no pain, and plantar fasciitis and heel pain with no heel spurs, though they often come together. Plantar fasciitis was thought for a number of years to cause heel spur formation, but a 2007 study (Li and Muehleman) presented a compelling argument against heel spur formation being caused by traction from the plantar aponeurosis and muscle attachments. By studying cadavers with heel spurs, including examining the direction of the spur bone fibers (*trabeculae*), the location of the spurs, and the variability of muscle and fiber attachments (or lack thereof) to the spur, they determined it was unlikely that heel spurs were formed by traction from these tissues pulling on the heel. Based on their findings, they hypothesized that heel spurs were more likely formed as a result of *vertical loading*, or pressure from above, and spurs actually serve the function of protecting the heel bone from developing micro fractures. They also noted a pattern of increasing number of heel spurs with age, and that for most people, heel stress would be a result of excessive force over a period of years, in addition to the individual variability in the arches and other foot structures. They also noted that, for non-athletes, increased *body mass index* (a measure of body fat based on the ratio of height and weight) plus a spur were two main factors in heel pain. If their hypothesis is correct, spurs would form in response to an increasing body mass, so gaining weight alone could account for both the heel pain and spur formation independently.

Stress Fractures

Several bones in the foot are susceptible to stress fractures, including the navicular, calcaneus (heel), and metatarsal bones. Symptoms may include pain that is worse during an activity, and possibly swelling and tenderness at the site of the fracture. You can probably still walk, and an X-ray might not necessarily be diagnostic, since stress fractures may not be visible on an X-ray. A bone scan or MRI might be necessary. Stress fractures are caused by prolonged, repeated loads such as running, hiking long distances, or being overweight. Tight calf and foot muscles are also likely involved, so the self-help techniques in this book will be helpful for preventing future injuries.

Foot Tendinopathies

There are numerous tendons in your foot that attach at various places, and allow you to flex and extend both your foot and toes. The most common symptom of foot tendinopathies is pain, though there may also be some swelling. A variety of problems can cause foot tendinopathies, including improper footwear, overuse, foot pronation, being overweight, and tight muscles in the calf and foot. The best way to resolve this problem is to wear proper shoes (addressed further in Appendix A), apply the self-help techniques found in this book to relieve muscle tightness, and if necessary, lose weight.

Claw Toes, Hammertoes, and Mallet Toe

These conditions are associated with long-standing tightness of the toe *long extensor* muscles (chapter 16), and often tight calf muscles too. With all three conditions, your toes are bent up at one of the toe's joints. A person with claw toe (or claw foot) also has a high arch, giving the foot a claw-like appearance. Self-help techniques may give at least partial relief, and proper footwear is essential to prevent further aggravation and deformity.

Bunions and Hallux Valgus

Hallux valgus is a painful condition where the big toe becomes displaced and deformed. Tightness and trigger points in the *flexor hallucis longus* muscle (chapter 15) can help cause hallux valgus, and the more the bone has spread, the more force is exerted by the muscle on the bone, making the cycle self-perpetuating. The *flexor hallucis brevis*, *adductor hallucis* and *abductor hallucis* (the superficial intrinsic foot muscles, chapter 17) become weak, allowing even further spread. A *bunion*, or swelling of the protective lubricating pad on the side of the big toe, can form and cause additional pain.

It is important to avoid high heels during childhood and teenage bone-formative years since this can drastically reduce the likelihood of developing bunions later in life. Relief of trigger points may stop the progression or even reverse some of the spread of hallux valgus and subsequent bunions, though surgery may be necessary if the condition has progressed far enough. Proper footwear and orthotics are essential if you have either of these conditions.

Toe Drop

Toe drop is caused by trigger points in the *tibialis anterior* muscle. You aren't able to lift your foot up when walking (plantar-flexion) and you can trip or fall. Trigger points can be caused by acute injuries or walking up or down hills when you aren't used to non-level surfaces. See chapter 14 for treatment of this condition.

Chapter 2: Locating and Treating Trigger Points: General Guidelines

Where to Start?

Chapter 3 contains the *Trigger Point Location Guide;* this will help you figure out which muscles in this book may harbor trigger points that might be causing your symptoms. Locate your pain or other symptoms for each area, and then refer to the chapters listed.

Each muscle chapter has drawings that show the most common pain referral areas for each trigger point. The more solid black or white area indicates the primary area of referral, which is almost always present, and the lighter stippled area shows the most likely secondary areas of referral, which may or may not be present. Keep in mind that the referral patterns only show the most *common* referral patterns; your referral pattern may be somewhat different or even completely different. You may also have overlapping referral patterns from trigger points in multiple muscles. These areas may be more extensive than the patterns common for individual muscles, and pain may be more intense. For this reason, over time, be sure to search for trigger points in all the muscles that refer pain to that area.

Each muscle chapter contains an anatomical drawing of the muscle or muscles covered in that chapter, with "X"'s showing some of the most common locations of trigger points. *There may be additional trigger points or they may be in different places, so search the entire muscle.*

Each muscle chapter also includes lists of common symptoms and factors that may cause or perpetuate trigger points. Again, these are only the most common; you may experience different symptoms, and your causes and perpetuating factors may be different. If you think you might have trigger points in a certain muscle but don't see any perpetuating factors that apply to you, try to imagine whether anything in your life is similar to something on the list that could be causing the same type of stress on the muscle.

Once you've determined which two muscles most closely fit your pain referral pattern and symptoms, start doing the self-help pressure and stretching, and eliminate the applicable perpetuating factors. Over the next several weeks, search for trigger points in additional muscles, and add those into your treatment regime as needed. As you start to feel better, you'll develop a clearer picture of which trigger points are causing your pain, and which perpetuating factors are reactivating your trigger points.

Other Things to Consider…

When you apply pressure to the trigger point, you can often reproduce the referred pain or other symptoms, but being unable to reproduce the referred pain or other symptoms by applying pressure does *not* rule out involvement of that specific trigger point. Try treating the trigger points that could be causing the problem anyway, and if you improve, even temporarily, assume that one of the trigger points you worked on is indeed at least part of the problem. For this reason, don't work on all the possible trigger points in one session, since you won't know which trigger point treated actually gave you relief.

Be aware that a *primary*, or *key*, trigger point can cause a *satellite* trigger point to develop in a different muscle. The satellite trigger point may have formed for one of these reasons: it lies within the referral zone of the primary trigger point, or it's in a muscle that is either substituting for, or is countering tension for the muscle that contains the primary trigger point. When doing self-treatments, be aware that if some of your trigger points are satellite trigger points, you won't get lasting relief until the primary trigger points have been treated. This is why it is important to work in the direction of referral (see "Do's" below).

You also need to be aware that central sensitization (explained in Appendix B) can cause the referral pattern to deviate from the most common pattern found in each muscle chapter. It may also cause trigger points in several muscles within a region to refer pain to the same area, making it more difficult to determine trigger point locations. This means you can't absolutely rule out the role of a potential trigger point based *only* on consideration of common referral patterns, since other factors may cause you to have an *uncommon* referral pattern. The more intense the earlier pain, the more intense the emotions associated with it, and the longer pain has lasted, the more likely central sensitization will cause deviation from the most common referral patterns.

A small percentage of people will get worse before they get better, mostly in complex cases. Or the pain may move around, or you may have the perception that the pain moved around only because the most painful areas have improved and now you are noticing the next most painful area more. I've only had a few cases where I wasn't able to help patients, because they were so frustrated after receiving little or no help from professional after professional that they only allowed me to treat them a few times before giving up, *even if they had improved*. If you get a little worse before you get better, you may be inclined to give up in the initial stages of treatment. I encourage you to give any treatment you try some amount of time before you decide it isn't working, even if your condition initially gets worse.

General Guidelines for Applying Self-Pressure

DON'Ts:

- **Do not apply pressure over varicose veins, open wounds, infections, herniated/bulging disks, areas of phlebitis/thrombophlebitis, or where clots are present or could be present. If you are pregnant, do not apply pressure on your legs.**

- **Most importantly: *Don't overdo the self-help techniques!*** Many people think that if some feels great, more will be even better, but you can actually make yourself worse by not following the guidelines. Expect gradual improvement, though you may improve most quickly during the initial weeks of therapy.

DO's:

- **Use a tennis ball, racquetball, golf ball, dog play ball, or baseball, or use your elbow or hand if instructed for particular muscles.** For balls, use the weight of your body to give you the pressure; don't press your back or limb onto the balls. The muscle you are working on should be as passive as possible. Use one ball at a time on your back, not one on each side.

- **Apply pressure for a minimum of eight seconds, and a maximum of one minute;** less than eight seconds may activate trigger points, and more than a minute will cut off the circulation for too long and make it worse. Time yourself first to be sure you are actually counting seconds at the correct speed.

- **It should be somewhat uncomfortable, or "hurt good," but it should not be so painful that you are either tensing up or holding your breath. If it is too painful, use a smaller or softer ball, or move to a softer surface (like a bed, or pad your surface with a pillow or blanket).** If it does *not* hurt at all, keep looking for tender spots, or try moving to a harder surface. If it's too tender to lie on, try putting a ball in a long sock and leaning against the wall. I only recommend using the wall if you cannot lie on the ball, since you are then using the very muscles you are trying to work on. You may need to use a combination of surfaces depending on the tenderness of different areas. Over time, as sensitivity decreases, you may need to change ball dimensions and/or hardness, or move to a harder surface.

- **Search the *entire* muscle for tender points, particularly the points of maximum tenderness.** Use the pictures to make sure you are getting the entire muscle and not just the worst spot. Many times a tendon attachment will hurt because the tight muscle is pulling on it, but if you don't treat the bulk of the muscle, it will keep pulling on the attachment.

- **Be sure to work on both sides of the body to keep the muscles balanced, but spend more time on the areas that need it more.** Except for very new one-sided injuries, the same muscle on the opposite side will almost always be tender with pressure, even if it has not yet started causing symptoms. If you loosen one side but not the other, it can lead to additional problems. Sometimes problems with the muscles on the opposite side are actually causing the symptoms, so it is always worth working on both sides.

- **Work in the direction of referral.** For example, if your outer leg muscles hurt and the pain is being referred from trigger points in the *gluteus minimus* muscle in the hip area, work on the hip area first, then the outer leg area.

- If you have limited time, **do one area thoroughly rather than rushing through many areas**. You are more likely to aggravate trigger points rather than inactivate them if you rush.

- **Do stretches *after* the trigger point work.** If you only have time to do one thing, do the ball/pressure work and skip the stretches.

- **Most people should work on their muscles one time per day initially.** If you have an appointment with your therapist, do not do your self-help the same day. If you are sore from your therapy appointment or your self-help, skip a day. If you are sore for more than one day or your symptoms get worse, it is likely that either the pressure was too hard or you held points for too long. Review these guidelines if that is the case. Tell your therapist if you are sore from their work. This is *not* a case of where if some is great, more is better.

  Pick a time when you will remember to do your self-help, i.e., when you wake up, when you watch television, or when you go to bed, and keep your balls by the bed (*but do not fall asleep on a ball!*).

  After a few weeks, you may wish to increase your self-help to twice per day, as long as you are not getting sore. If a particular activity bothers you, you may wish to do the self-help before and after the activity. If you start getting sore or your symptoms get worse, decrease your self-help frequency.

  Treat your trigger points for as long as they are sensitive, even if active symptoms have disappeared. If trigger points are still tender, they are *latent*, and could easily be reactivated. Most likely you will start forgetting as symptoms disappear; however, the most important thing you will have learned is what to do if your symptoms return.

- **If you have questions or your symptoms get worse, or you are sore for more than one day, stop the self-help until you have had a chance to consult with your therapist.** They should be able to help you figure out any problems.

- **Take your balls on trips with you**, since travel frequently aggravates trigger points. You may even wish to keep some balls at work.

General Guidelines for Stretches and Conditioning

It is very important to distinguish the difference between *stretching* and *conditioning* exercises. *Stretching* means you gently lengthen the muscle fibers. *Conditioning* means you are trying to strengthen the muscle. Doctors Travell and Simons found that *active* trigger points benefited from stretching, but were usually aggravated by conditioning exercises. Once trigger points have been *inactivated*, conditioning is beneficial. Make sure your physical therapist or physiotherapist is familiar with trigger points, and begins your therapy with stretching exercises.

Usually two weeks of trigger point self-help treatment will be sufficient before adding in conditioning exercises, but if your trigger points are still very irritable, you will need to wait until your symptoms improve. Meanwhile, learn the stretches in this book. If you are not sure whether an assigned activity is a stretch or conditioning, ask your practitioner. I will not cover guidelines for conditioning exercises in depth here, since your physical therapist or physiotherapist will prescribe them.

DON'Ts:

- **Don't bounce on stretches, and avoid stretching when your muscles are tired or cold.**

- **Don't do a conditioning exercise just because it worked for someone else.** Doctors Travell and Simons said "Exercise should be regarded as a prescription, much as one prescribes medication. Like a drug, there is a right kind, dose, and timing of exercise." Often a friend will recommend an exercise that worked for them, but you are a different person with a different set of symptoms, and you should no more do their assigned exercises than you would take their prescribed medications. Be sure to tell your therapist all of the activities and exercises/stretches you are doing, because one of these can be contributing to your trigger point activation.

- **Don't keep doing an exercise or stretch that is aggravating your symptoms.** Check with your therapist to determine why it is bothering you and to find out how to proceed.

DO's:

- **Stretch slowly, and only to the point of just getting a gentle stretch; *don't force it.*** If you stretch the muscles too hard or too fast, you can aggravate trigger points.

- **Hold your stretch for 30 to 60 seconds.** There will be little benefit after 30 seconds, but it will not hurt you to stretch for longer either. You may repeat the stretch after releasing and breathing.

- **For any type of repetitive exercise, breathe and rest between each cycle of the exercise.**

- **If you are sore for more than one day** from exercises or stretches, reduce the number of repetitions and try again after the soreness has disappeared. If you are still sore for two days after the exercise or stretch, it needs to be changed.

General Guidelines for Muscle Care

These are some general suggestions for taking care of your muscles; each muscle chapter will have specific suggestions.

DON'Ts:

- Never put the maximum load on a muscle -- it is too easy to strain it.

- Don't lift something too heavy -- ask for help.

- Don't keep muscles in positions of sustained contractions, where you are holding them tense or in sustained use. In order to increase blood flow and bring oxygen and nutrients to the muscles, they need to alternately constrict and relax.

- Don't sit for too long in one position.

- Don't expose your muscles to cold drafts.

DO's:

- After treatments, gently use the muscle in a normal way that uses its full range-of-motion, but avoid strenuous activities immediately afterward or until the trigger points aren't so easily aggravated, whichever is longer.

- Vary your activities so you are not doing any one thing for too long. Rest and take breaks frequently from any given activity.

- Lift with your knees bent and your back straight, with the object close to your chest.

- Notice where you hold tension and practice relaxing those areas.

- Swimming is generally a good exercise, and bicycling is easier on the body than running, but in both cases, take care to avoid straining the *trapezius* and neck muscles. A recumbent, stationary, or other bike that allows you to sit more upright is preferable.

- When starting an exercise program, *underestimate* what you will be able to do. Gradually add increments in duration, rate, and effort, and in amounts that will not cause you to be sore or activate trigger points.

- Warm-up adequately for sports activities.

- If you are working with a practitioner, they should be able to help you prioritize what needs to be done in order of most importance. If your practitioner is giving you too many things to do at once, be sure to tell them that you are overwhelmed and need to set priorities. Giving a patient too many assignments is all too easy for a practitioner to do, especially when they are first out of school and brimming with many useful ideas and suggestions.

Be sure to return to this chapter often to review the guidelines to ensure you are treating the muscles properly, particularly if something is not working for you, or trigger points are getting aggravated instead of inactivated. Chances are you have forgotten to follow these guidelines.

Be sure to set realistic goals. Focus on a few muscles at a time unless there is a reason that you need to work on several together. Setting unrealistic goals can discourage you, and cause you to give up. It's better to pick just a few things and do them well rather than rush through too many self-help techniques or suggestions and do them poorly. You probably won't be able to apply pressure on five different muscles and stretch them, get orthotics and replace bad shoes, change your diet, and start walking every day all in the first week. Pace yourself so that this is an enjoyable process, and work on the perpetuating factors over time.

Chapter 3: Trigger Point Location Guide

To figure out which muscles to work on first, look at the trigger point location guides and refer to the chapters listed for each. Examine the photos of referral patterns in each chapter and try to find those that most closely match your pain pattern, and read the list of symptoms for each muscle. Refer to chapter 2 for additional instructions on locating and treating trigger points, and general guidelines for applying pressure, stretching, and general muscle care.

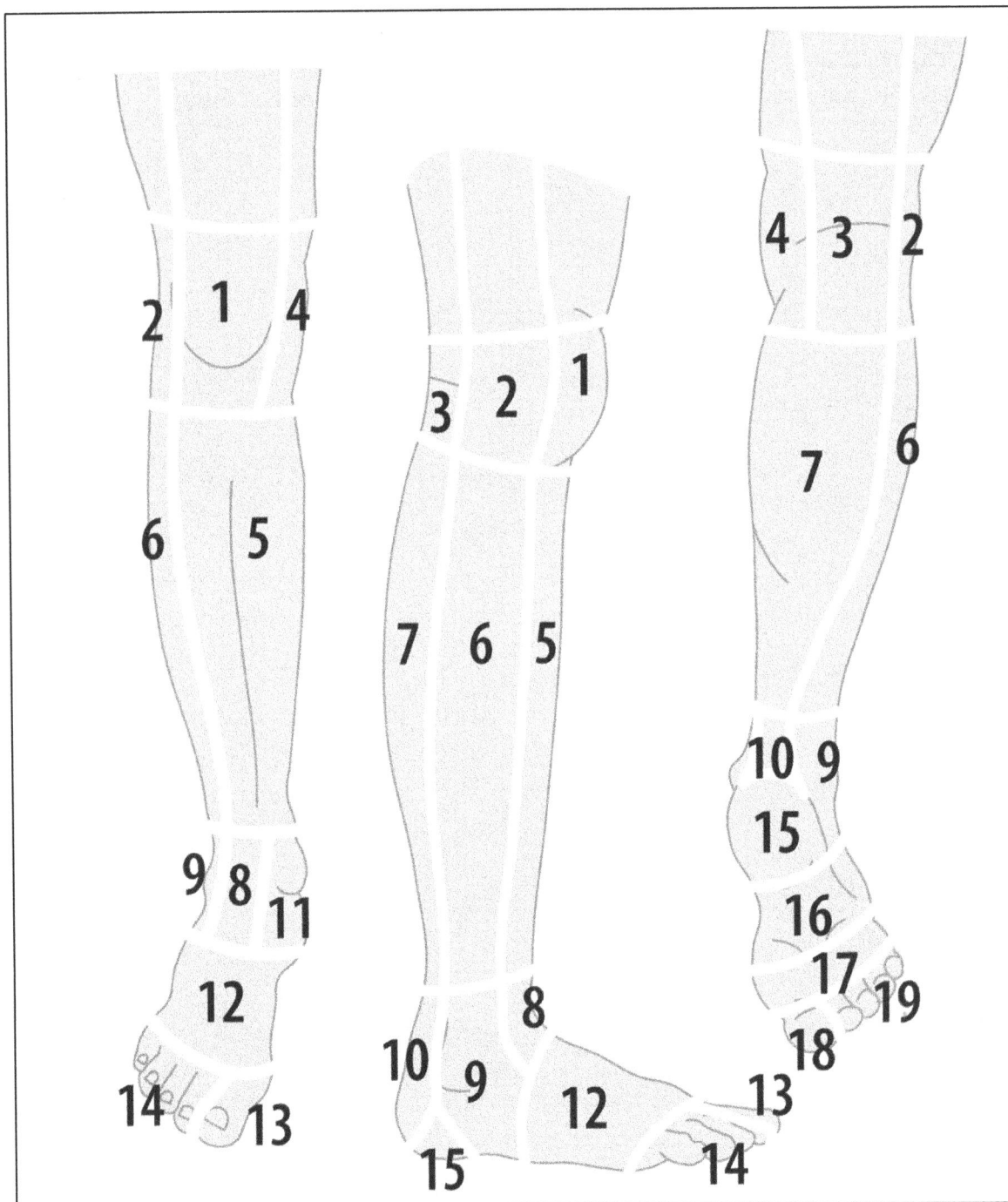

1. Quadriceps Femoris Muscles (5)
   Adductors Longus & Brevis (6)

2. Vastus Lateralis (5)

3. Gastrocnemius (10)
   Hamstring Muscles (8)
   Popliteus (9)
   Soleus (11)

4. Quadriceps Femoris Muscles (5)
   Adductor Muscles of the Hip (6)
   Sartorius (7)

5. Tibialis Anterior (14)
   Adductors Longus & Brevis (6)

6. Gastrocnemius (10)
   Gluteus Minimus (4)
   Peroneus Longus & Brevis (13)
   Vastus Lateralis (5)

7. Soleus (11)
   Gastrocnemius (10)
   Gluteus Minimus (4)
   Semimembranosus & Semitendinosus (8)
   Flexor Digitorum Longus (15)
   Tibialis Posterior (12)

8. Tibialis Anterior (14)
   Peroneus Tertius (13)
   Long Extensor Muscles of the Toes (16)

9. Peroneal Muscles (13)

10. Soleus (11)
    Tibialis Posterior (12)

11. Abductor Hallucis (17)
    Flexor Digitorum Longus (15)

12. Extensors Digitorum Brevis and Hallucis Brevis (17)
    Long Extensor Muscles of the Toes (16)
    Deep Intrinsic Foot Muscles (18)
    Tibialis Anterior (14)

13. Tibialis Anterior (14)
    Extensor Hallucis Longus (16)
    Flexor Hallucis Brevis (18)

14. Foot Interossei (18)
    Extensor Digitorum Longus (16)

15. Soleus (11)
    Quadratus Plantae (18)
    Abductor Hallucis (17)
    Tibialis Posterior (12)

16. Gastrocnemius (10)
    Flexor Digitorum Longus (15)
    Deep Intrinsic Foot Muscles (18)
    Soleus (11)
    Abductor Hallucis (17)
    Tibialis Posterior (12)

17. Deep Intrinsic Foot Muscles (18)
    Superficial Intrinsic Foot Muscles (17)
    Long Flexor Muscles of the Toes (15)
    Tibialis Posterior (12)

18. Flexor Hallucis Longus (15)
    Flexor Hallucis Brevis (18)
    Tibialis Posterior (12)

19. Flexor Digitorum Longus (15)
    Tibialis Posterior (12)

Muscle chapters for all of the remaining areas of the body can be found in *Pain Relief with Trigger Point Self-Help.* Please see the end of this book for more information.

Blank Body Chart

You may wish to make copies of the following blank body chart and draw your symptom pattern on one of them with a colored marker. Then you can compare your pattern with the pain referral pictures in chapters 4 through 18. Out to the side of each painful area, note your pain intensity on a scale of 1 to 10 and the percent of time you feel pain in that area—for example, 6.5/80%. (If you are unable to print from your device, go to http://triggerpointrelief.com/pain_guides.html for a copy you can print off.)

I recommend that you fill out a body chart at least a couple of times per week. Date them so that you'll be able to keep them in order. This chronological record will come in handy in several ways. It will:

- make it easier for you to discern which patterns fit your pain referral most closely;
- help you recognize the factors that cause and perpetuate your symptoms by matching fluctuations in the level and frequency of your symptoms;
- allow you to track your progress (or lack thereof) and provide a historical record of any injuries.

As your condition improves, you may forget how intense your symptoms were originally, and you may think you're not getting any better. You'll be able to see that you are improving, even if you have an occasional setback. One thing to note, however, is that not everyone can accurately draw their pain location, due in part to lack of familiarity with anatomy, so take that possibility into consideration and check muscles with adjacent referral patterns just in case your drawing is inaccurate.

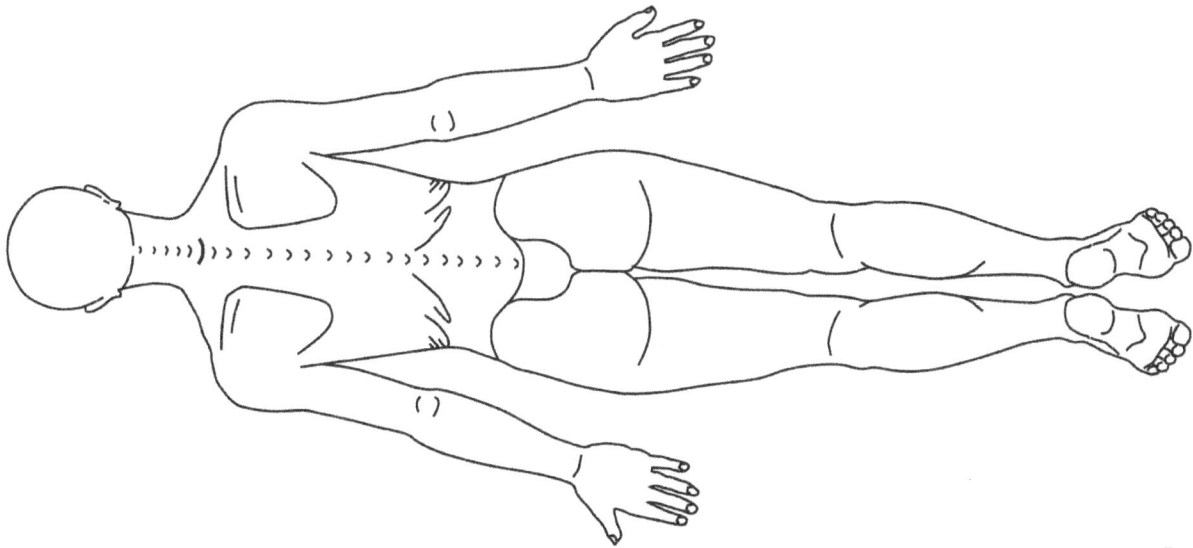

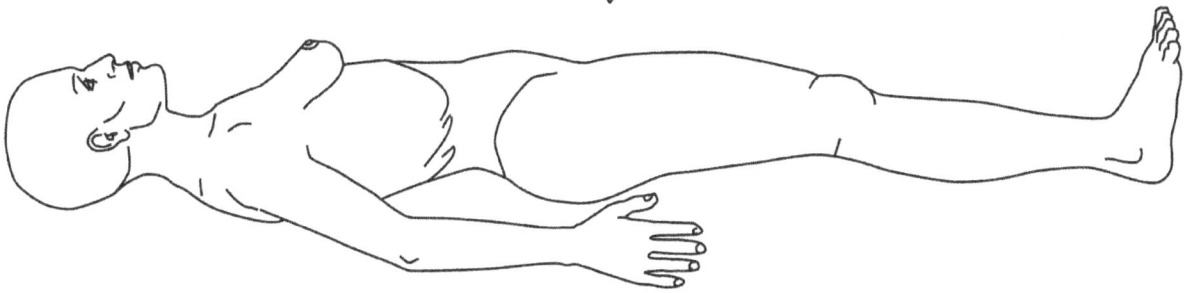

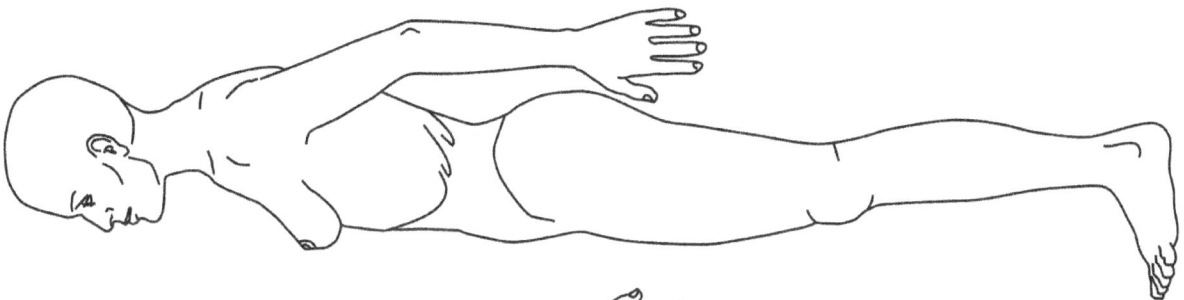

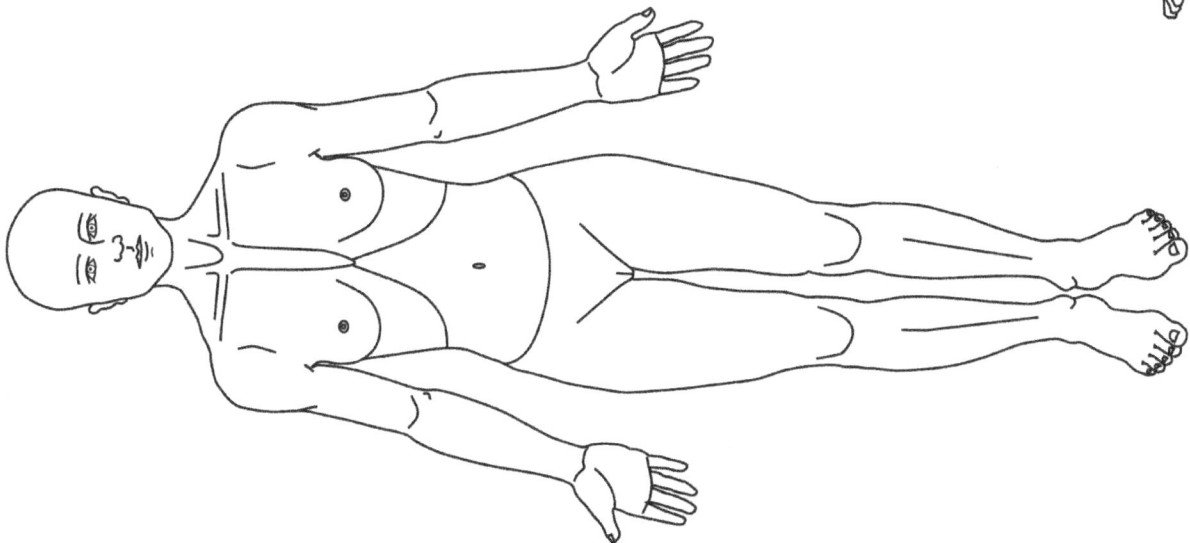

Chapter 4: Gluteus Minimus

Referred pain from trigger points in the *gluteus minimus* frequently gets diagnosed by both patients and practitioners as "sciatic pain," because of the distribution pattern down the side and back of the legs. At least 80% of pain down the leg comes from trigger point referral, not from "pinched nerves," a herniated disc, or stenosis in a lumbar vertebra (narrowing of either the big hole in the vertebra that the spinal cord goes through, or narrowing of the smaller holes the nerves travel out through). Since "sciatica" is usually assumed to be caused by compression of a nerve, pain referrals from trigger points are probably more aptly called "pseudo-sciatica."

I have found that if the pain is truly coming from a disc or problem with a lumbar vertebra, the patient usually draws a referral pattern that starts as a thin line coming from a very specific spot on one side of a lumbar vertebra, and then continues into the gluteal area and down the leg. The pain is usually sharper and intense. If the pain referral starts in the gluteal area and not a pinpoint spot in the lumbar area, it is likely caused by trigger points in either the *gluteus minimus* or *piriformis* muscles. If it does start next to a vertebra, you need to see a health care provider and get an MRI to be evaluated for disc problems and stenosis.

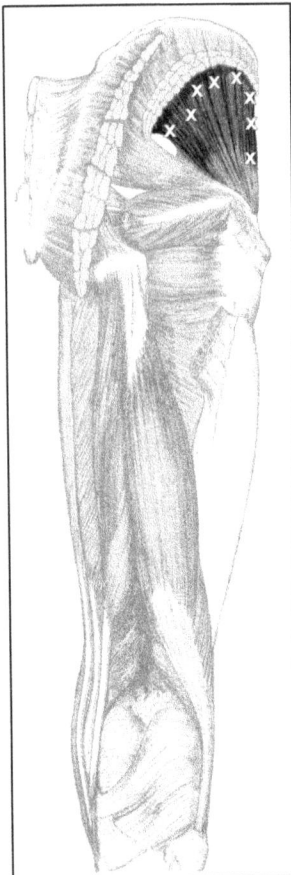

Back view of gluteal area and thigh

Common Symptoms

- the anterior portion of the muscle (on your side, under the seam of your pants) refers pain down the side of the leg to the ankle, and possibly to a spot on the backside of your buttocks
- the posterior portion of the muscle is part way between the side and the backside, and refers pain over the gluteal area and down the back of the leg into the calf
- hip pain may cause a limp with walking
- pain with sleeping on the affected side, severe enough to wake you
- difficulty rising out of a chair after sitting for a while
- difficulty in finding a comfortable position standing, walking, or lying down
- pain with running or hiking

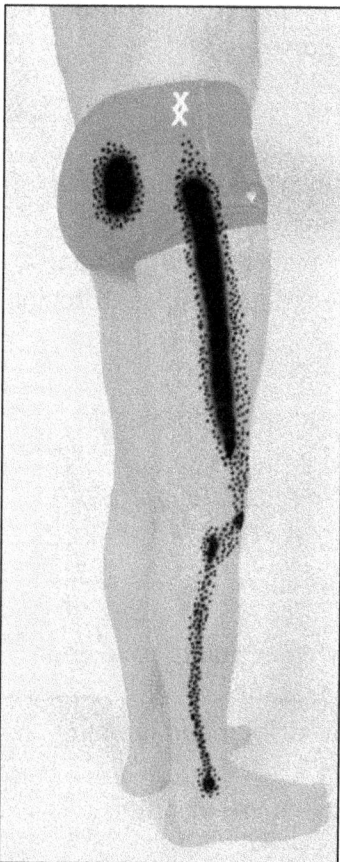

Gluteus Minimus Anterior   **Gluteus Minimus Posterior**

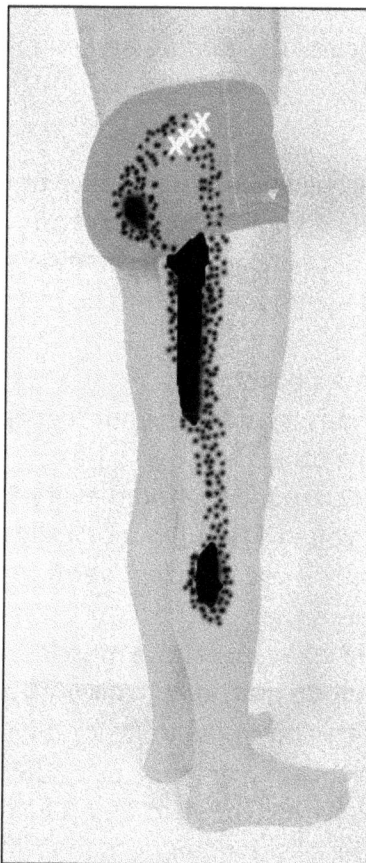

Causes and Perpetuation of Trigger Points

- sudden or chronic overuse
- sitting with a wallet in your back pocket
- standing for long periods with your weight shifted to one side or with your feet too close together
- sitting for too long, especially when driving
- a fall

- walking or running too far or too fast, especially on rough ground
- overuse while playing tennis, racquetball, or handball
- chilling of the muscle or the body as a whole
- walking with a limp from an injury
- injections of medications, especially irritants, can cause pain that lasts for months
- the sacroiliac joint out-of-alignment (the joint where the sacrum and big pelvic bone join)
- a nerve root irritation
- a small hemipelvis (either the right or left half of the pelvis)
- obesity tends to overload these muscles

This is a list of perpetuating factors specific only to trigger points in this *muscle. For a full list of perpetuating factors that can cause and perpetuate trigger points anywhere in the body and which also apply to this muscle, please see "Appendix A" (found at the end of this book), since some may need to be addressed for lasting pain relief.*

Helpful Hints

- Runners and avid hikers usually have *gluteus minimus* trigger points. If you have located trigger points with the self-help techniques, back off on your runs or hikes until the trigger points have improved dramatically. You can then *slowly* increase your mileage, staying out of the pain zone. I recommend doing the ball self-work and ample stretching before and after the run.
- Don't carry a wallet in your back pocket.
- If you must stand for long periods, stand with your feet apart and shift your weight frequently from one foot to the other.
- If you sit for long periods, move around the room every 15-20 minutes. A timer set across the room ensures that you will get up periodically to turn it off.
- Keep your body, and particularly these muscles, warm.
- Sleep with a pillow between your legs.
- If you are obese, don't over-do exercising these muscles until trigger points have been inactivated and strength is built-up gradually. Walk with a wider stance.
- See a chiropractor or osteopathic physician to check the sacroiliac joint and lumbar vertebrae for alignment problems.
- If you have a small hemipelvis (either the right or left half of the pelvis) or other structural imbalance, see a specialist for compensating lifts and pads.
- Acupuncture will help with disc problems, but will only help with the pain from stenosis. It will not affect the stenosis, which may require surgery. These surgeries have gotten very sophisticated in recent years, and usually have you back on your feet the day after the surgery.
- If you receive muscular injections, avoid this muscle. Inject into the *gluteus medius* and *deltoid* muscles, since they are less prone to developing trigger points.
- If pain remains after a laminectomy surgery, check the *gluteus minimus* for trigger points.

Self-Help Techniques

Applying Pressure

Gluteus Minimus Pressure: Be sure to work on the *gluteus minimus* muscles on both right *and* left sides of your body. Common trigger points in the *gluteus minimus* are found in the upper third of the back of your gluteal area, to over on the side between your hip joint and the top of your pelvis.

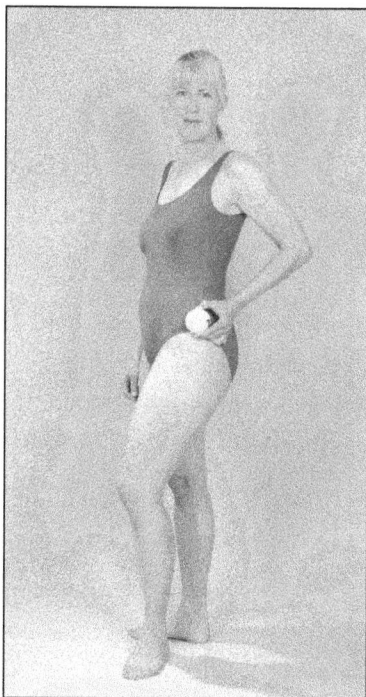

Gluteus Minimus Anterior
Demonstrating location to use ball

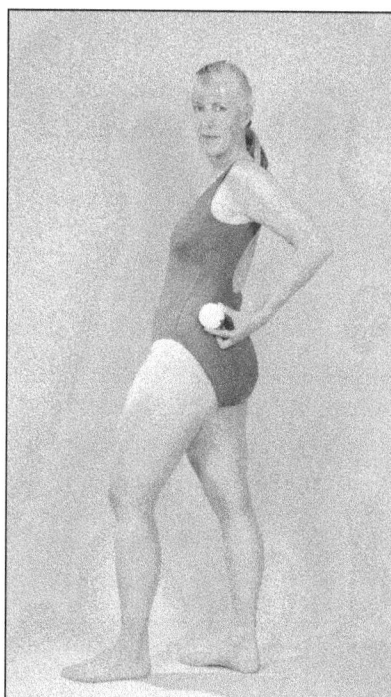

Gluteus Minimus Posterior
Demonstrating location to use ball

Lying face-up on a tennis ball, move the ball with your hand while searching for trigger points.

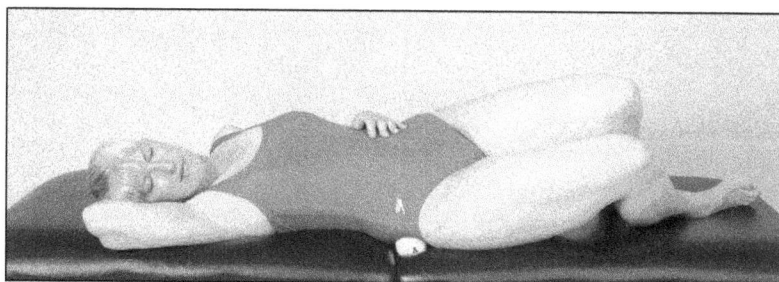

Start moving gradually out onto your side. By the time you work on the entire *gluteus minimus* muscle, you will be lying on your side. Many patients make the mistake of not getting far enough forward. If you are working over the seam of your pants, you are reaching all the points; otherwise, keep searching further forward.

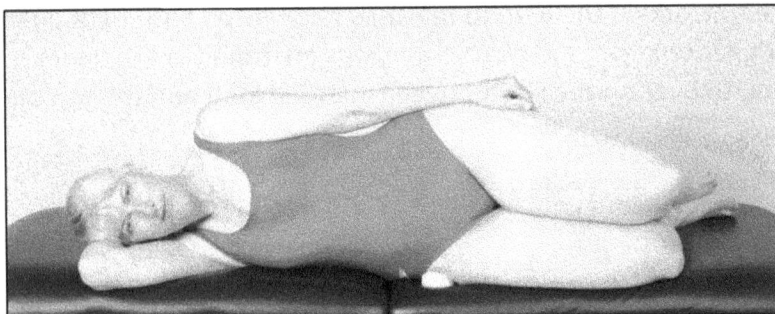

Stretches

Gluteus Minimus Stretch, Anterior Muscle Portion: To stretch the *anterior* fibers of the *gluteus minimus* muscle, lie on your side on the edge of the bed with your back flush to the edge. Allow your top leg to drop behind you, off the edge. Allow gravity to give you a stretch. If you want more of a stretch, put the heel of your opposite leg on the side of your calf. Then move your heel closer to your knee for an even greater stretch.

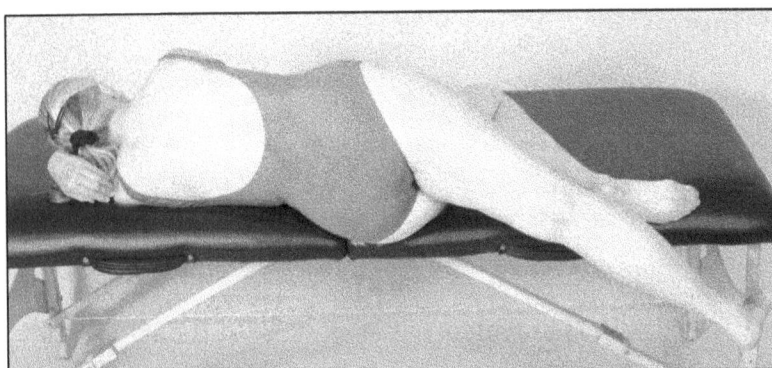

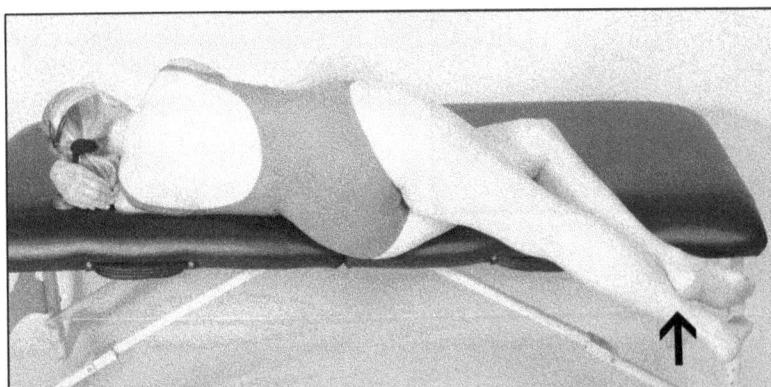

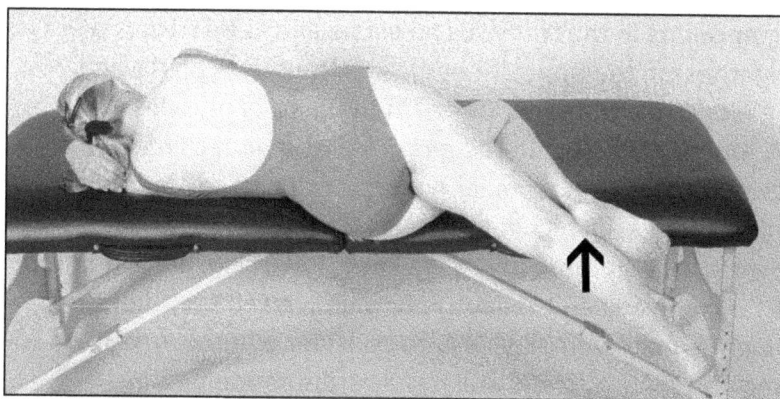

Gluteus Minimus Stretch, Posterior Muscle Portion: To stretch the *posterior* fibers of the *gluteus minimus* muscle, lie on your side and position yourself at the foot of the bed with the top leg out over the end and slightly forward of the line of your trunk, with your toes slightly rotated toward the floor. Your bottom leg is bent at more than 90°, so that it is still mostly on the bed. Let gravity give you a stretch.

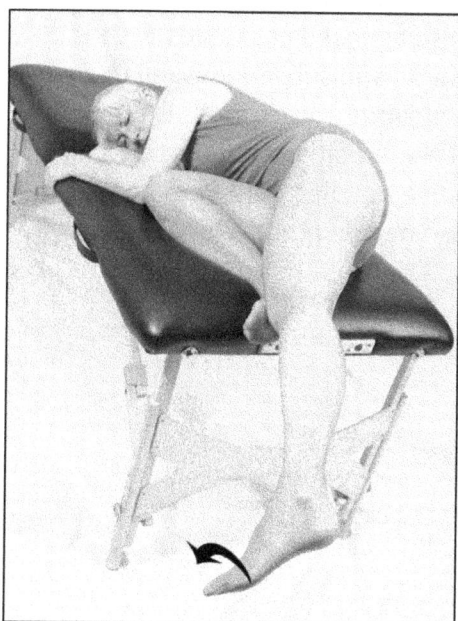

Also See:

*   Vastus lateralis (chapter 5)
*   Peroneus longus (chapter 13)

If the pain feels deep in the hip joint, it is more likely coming from trigger points in the *tensor fasciae latae* muscle instead of the *gluteus minimus*. If pain is over the sacrum (the bony triangle between the spine and the tailbone) or the sacroiliac joint, trigger points are more likely located in the *gluteus medius*.

If you only get temporary relief with the self-help techniques, you may need to check the *quadratus lumborum*, since trigger points in that muscle can cause and keep trigger points in the *gluteus minimus* activated. Tightness in the opposite *paraspinal* muscles can tilt and rotate the pelvis, causing pain in the hip joint and trigger points in the *gluteal* muscles

You may also need to search for trigger points in the *piriformis* and *gluteus maximus*, since trigger points in those muscles can either cause similar pain referral patterns or may affect or be affected by *gluteus minimus* trigger points in some way.

Since trigger points in these muscles don't directly cause knee, lower leg, ankle and foot pain, they are not addressed in this book. If you can't relieve your pain with the self-help techniques in this book after six to eight weeks, you may wish to consider whether you need to treat trigger points in these additional muscles, or if you still have perpetuating factors to resolve. Go to the end of this book for other books by the author that provide self-treatment techniques of muscles not covered in this book.

Differential Diagnosis: If the pain is very localized over the hip joint or perhaps from the buttocks down the side to the knee, it may be trochanteric bursitis, which is inflammation of a fluid-filled sack over the bone that allows the *gluteus minimus* tendon to glide over the bony prominence. The hip joint will be very tender to pressure, and applying pressure reproduces the symptoms. *Gluteus minimus* trigger points can also be misdiagnosed as bursitis, so it is always worth checking the surrounding muscles for trigger points and subsequent relief. Since, in every case of *true* bursitis that I have treated, the *gluteus minimus* muscle was also tight, I suspect tightness and trigger points are a causative factor for the bursitis. Acupuncture can treat bursitis: I lay the patient on their side and place four to five needles around the bursa and one in the center, which is called *"surround the dragon."* I also needle points along the gallbladder meridian, in addition to any trigger points that are contributing to the irritation of the bursa.

Chapter 5: Quadriceps Femoris Muscle Group

(Rectus Femoris, Vastus Medialis, Vastus Intermedius, Vastus Lateralis)

Trigger points in the *quadriceps femoris* muscle group are very common and frequently overlooked, mainly because they only minimally restrict range-of-motion, if at all.

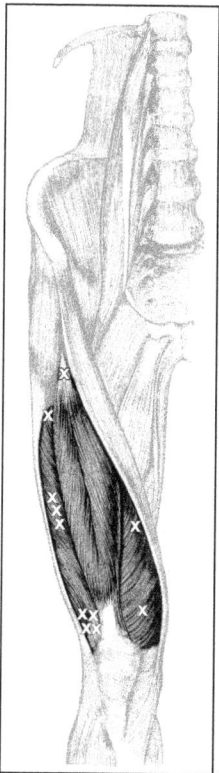

Front view of thigh

Common Symptoms

- referred pain on your thigh and knee, and possibly down the outside of your lower leg
- see the pictures (below) for all the trigger points and associated referral patterns
- if you have weakness when extending your knee, you probably have either active or latent trigger points in the *rectus femoris, vastus medialis,* and/or *vastus intermedius*

Rectus Femoris
- pain deep in your knee, in and around your kneecap, and possibly on the front of your thigh at night in bed
- even though the pain is in the knee area, the trigger point is just below the crease of your groin
- occasionally a trigger point will be found just above the knee, and will refer pain deep into your knee joint
- going down stairs is more likely to be a problem than going up stairs

- in above-knee amputees, phantom limb pain may come from trigger points in the *rectus femoris*, particularly if the muscle was stretched to cover the bone

Vastus Medialis
- the trigger point closer to the knee refers pain to the front of your knee, and the trigger point about mid-thigh refers pain over the inside of your knee and thigh
- toothache-like pain deep in the knee joint that can interrupt sleep, and may be mistaken for inflammation of the knee
- trigger points only minimally restrict range-of motion and may only affect leg function, rather than causing pain
- unexpected "buckling of the knee" (usually when walking on rough ground) produced by muscle weakness, which can lead to falls and injury
- if trigger points are found in both the *vastus medialis* and the *rectus femoris*, your hip may buckle

Vastus Intermedius
- intense pain at mid-thigh, closer to the outside of your thigh
- pain usually with movement, and rarely with rest
- difficulty fully straightening your knee which causes a limp when walking, especially after sitting for awhile
- difficulty with climbing stairs
- a "buckling knee" can be caused by a combination of trigger points in the *vastus intermedius* and the two heads of the *gastrocnemius* (chapter 10) below the crease on the back side of your knee
- trigger points can cause your kneecap to lock, though this is more common in the *vastus lateralis*
- this muscle is more difficult to find with your fingers since it is located underneath the *rectus femoris*

Vastus Lateralis
- the *vastus lateralis* develops multiple trigger points along the outside of the thigh, causing a variety of referral patterns along the outside of the thigh, knee, and possibly down into your calf
- pain with walking, and you may drag your foot on the affected side
- pain that disturbs your sleep when lying on the involved side
- a "stuck patella" (kneecap) that can cause difficulty in straightening or bending your knee after getting up from a chair
- if the kneecap is completely locked, your knee will be slightly bent and you cannot walk, or sit without the leg supported in the locked position
- going up stairs is more likely to be a problem than going down stairs
- trigger point referral can be mis-diagnosed as trochanteric bursitis if pain is referred over the outside of the hip bone (the greater trochanter)

Rectus femoris

Vastus Intermedius

Vastus medialis

Vastus medialis

Vastus lateralis

Vastus lateralis

Vastus lateralis

Vastus lateralis

Vastus lateralis

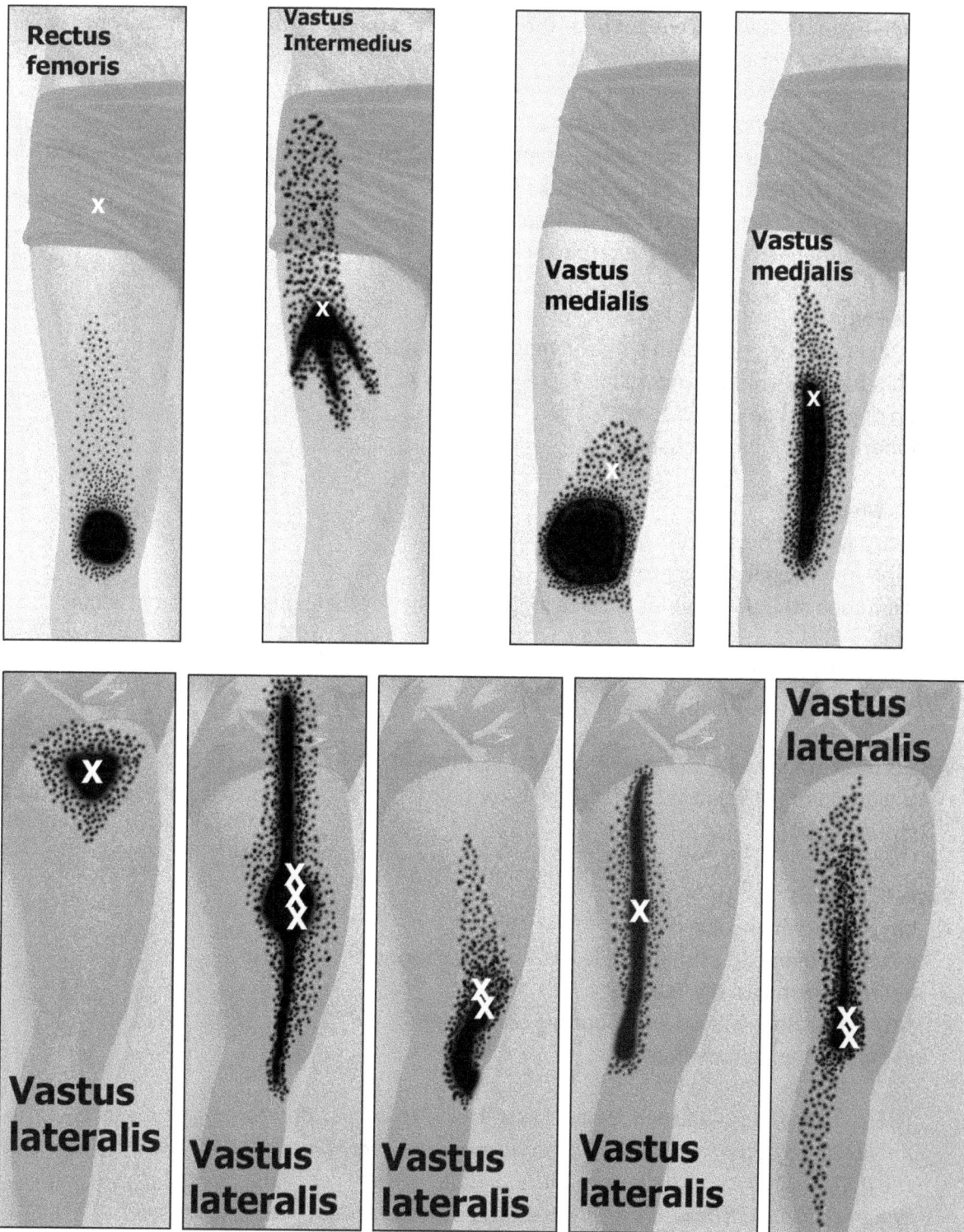

Causes and Perpetuation of Trigger Points

- stumbling, such as into a hole or off a curb
- sports injuries
- a direct blow to the front of the thigh
- deep knee bends

- knee extensions with a weight near the ankle (see a physical therapist for a proper way to do this exercise)
- any lengthy immobilization, such as wearing a cast on your leg
- tightness in the *hamstrings* (chapter 8)
- active trigger points in the *soleus* (chapter 11), which restrict the motion of the ankle and lead to overload of the *quadriceps femoris* group
- injections of drugs, such as insulin, into the thigh
- sitting with one foot under your buttocks

Rectus Femoris
- sitting for a long time with a heavy weight on your lap
- a hip fracture and/or surgery
- hip degenerative joint disease
- abnormal hip joint mechanics

Vastus Medialis
- excessive foot pronation
- flat feet (which leads to pronation)
- strenuous athletic activities such as jogging, skiing, football, basketball, and soccer
- a fall
- a direct trauma to the knee joint and/or muscle
- kneeling on a hard surface

Vastus Intermedius
- trigger points develop secondary to trigger points in the other muscles of the *quadriceps femoris* group

Vastus Lateralis
- hip degenerative joint disease
- a sudden overload of the muscle, such as with sports accidents
- a direct trauma to the muscle
- sitting for a long period with your leg out straight
- abnormal hip joint mechanics

This is a list of perpetuating factors specific only to trigger points in these muscles. For a full list of perpetuating factors that can cause and perpetuate trigger points anywhere in the body and which also apply to these muscles, please see "Appendix A" (found at the end of this book), since some may need to be addressed for lasting pain relief

Helpful Hints
- It is important to identify and treat any lumbar vertebrae out-of-alignment or hip alignment problems. See a chiropractor or osteopathic physician for evaluation and treatment.
- Get corrective orthotics to solve foot pronation problems.

- Don't wear high heels.
- Do not do deep knee bends or squats.
- When getting out of a chair, use your arms to assist you in rising.
- Avoid picking things up off the floor.
- Avoid sitting in the same position for extended periods of time, especially with your thighs at less than a 90-degree angle to your trunk. Be sure to use a lumbar support. Don't sit with your legs extended straight out in front of you. Sitting in a rocking chair helps keep the muscles mobilized.
- If you have trigger points in the *vastus medialis* or *vastus lateralis*, sleep on the unaffected side with a pillow between your legs. Don't bring your thighs up toward your chest, and don't straighten your legs out all the way either.
- Don't kneel for long periods of time. Sit on a low stool and take frequent breaks.
- When driving, use a lumbar support and something like a pillow under the buttocks to increase the angle between your torso and thigh. Take frequent breaks.
- Don't sit with your foot under your buttocks.
- If one leg is anatomically shorter than the other, see a specialist to get a compensating lift.
- In the initial stages of treatment, you may wish to wear a neoprene knee brace which will help remind you to be careful with your leg, and will maintain warmth around the lower ends of the muscles.
- A buckling knee can also be caused by anterior subluxation of the lateral tibial plateau, which requires surgical correction. But since trigger points in the *vastus medialis* are the more likely culprits, search that muscle first.
- Trigger points in the upper part of the *vastus lateralis* commonly get mis-diagnosed as trochanteric bursitis. See the *gluteus minimus* muscle (chapter 4) for more information on bursitis.

Self-Help Techniques

Also search for trigger points in the *gluteus minimus* (anterior portion, chapter 4) and the *tensor fasciae latae*, since they can have referral patterns similar to *vastus lateralis* trigger points. If pain is on the front or inside of your thigh, also search the *adductor* muscles of the hip (*adductors longus* and/or *brevis* and *gracilis*, chapter 6). You will also need to search the *hamstrings* (chapter 8) and *soleus* (chapter 11) muscles, since they can activate and perpetuate trigger points in the *quadriceps femoris* group. If you find trigger points in the *rectus femoris*, also search the others in the quadriceps group, and the *sartorius* (chapter 7) and *iliopsoas*. If you find trigger points in the *vastus medialis*, also search the *rectus femoris, peroneus longus* (chapter 13), *adductor* muscles of the hip (chapter 6), *tensor fasciae latae*, and *gluteus medius*. If you find trigger points in the *vastus intermedius*, also search the *rectus femoris* and *vastus lateralis*. If you find trigger points in the *vastus lateralis*, also search the *gluteus minimus* muscle (anterior portion, chapter 4). (See the end of this book for other books by the author that provide self-treatment techniques of muscles not covered in this book.)

Applying Pressure

Do not apply pressure to your legs if you have varicose veins in the area to be treated - - it could release a clot that could go to your heart or brain! *An acupuncturist or massage therapist should treat your legs, because they can avoid the veins.* You may still do the stretches and exercises below.

Hamstrings Pressure: Treat the *hamstrings* muscle group first (chapter 8), to avoid the cramping that can be caused by releasing the *quadriceps femoris* group. If you don't find trigger points in the *hamstrings*, you can probably skip this step in the future.

Vastus Lateralis Pressure: To work on the *vastus lateralis* muscle, start with the *gluteus minimus* (chapter 4) self-help ball work. Then continue on down the side of your thigh, using your hand to move the tennis ball as you search for tender points. Be sure to work the whole length of the muscle.

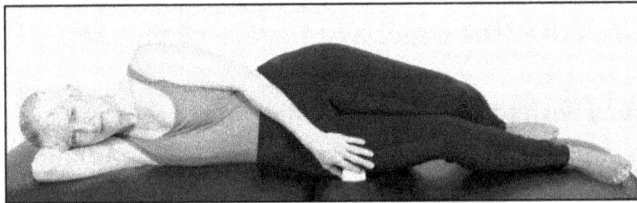

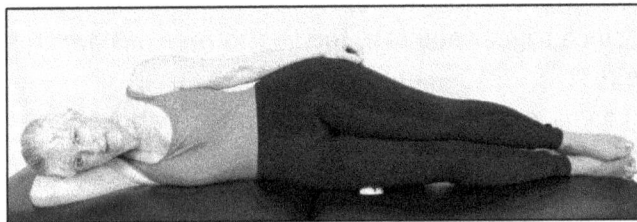

There may be some trigger points under the edge of the kneecap. Straighten out your leg, wrap your hands around your knee, and put both thumbs on the edge of the kneecap. Press the kneecap away from you while simultaneously pressing into trigger points in that area.

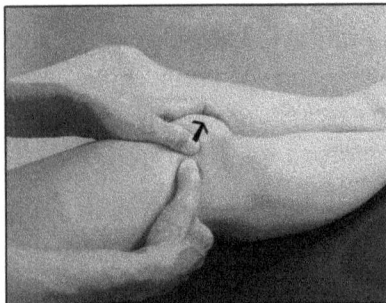

Rectus Femoris / Vastus Intermedius Pressure: To work on the *rectus femoris* and the underlying *vastus intermedius*, roll onto your stomach and with your leg bent, move the tennis ball around, checking for tender points. Be sure and work the entire length of the muscles.

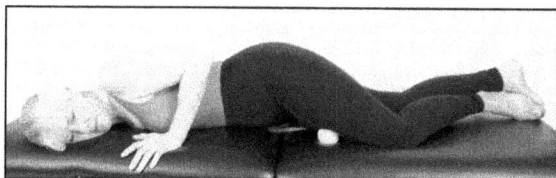

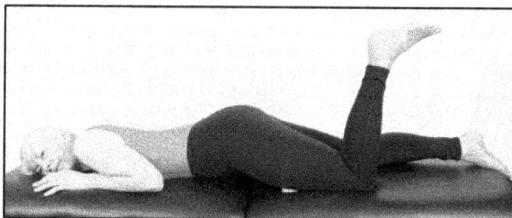

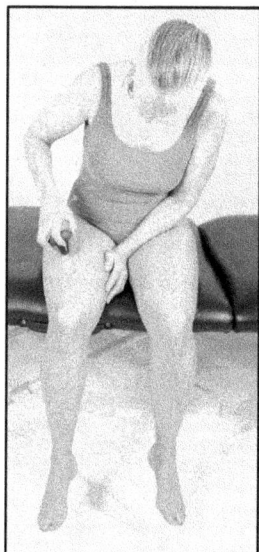

As an alternative, use a golf ball or other pressure device in the center of your palm, and press into tender points. This is less effective than laying on the ball due to the thickness of the *rectus femoris.*

Vastus Medialis Pressure: To work on the *vastus medialis*, use your thumb, or a golf ball or other pressure device held in the center of the palm of your opposite hand to press into tender points. It does not take a lot of pressure to treat these trigger points.

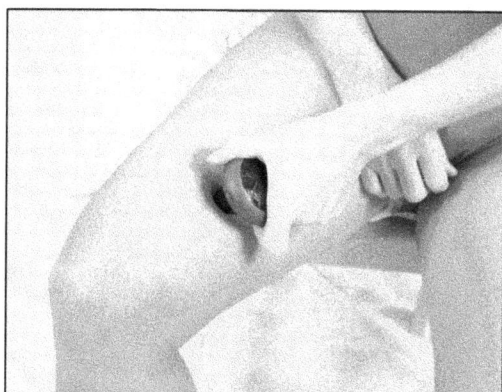

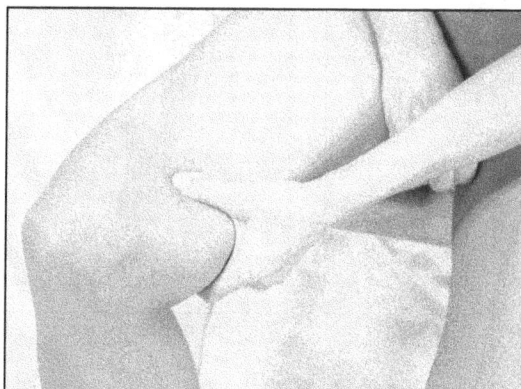

Stretches

Quadriceps Side-lying Stretch: Lying in bed on your side, bend your bottom leg to almost a 90° angle to the trunk, so you can rest your top knee on the bottom foot. Grab the ankle of your upper leg and pull it up behind you, so you are getting a stretch on the front of the thigh.

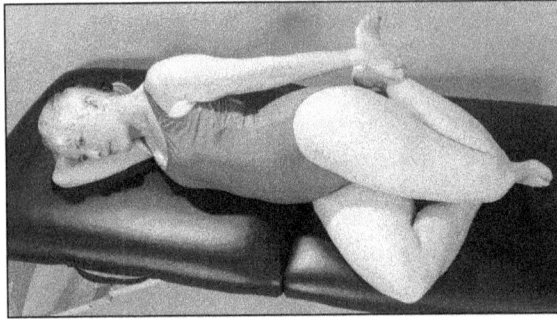

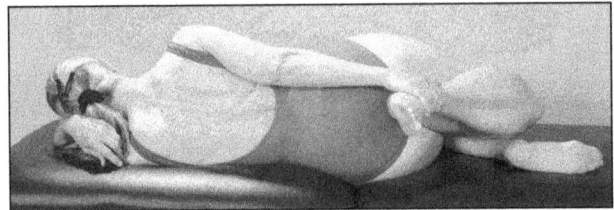

Quadriceps Standing Stretch: Hold onto a counter or other non-mobile piece of furniture for support. Grab your ankle using the hand on the same side, and pull your leg up behind you. Then with the *opposite* hand, grab the *same* ankle and pull your leg up behind you. The first part emphasizes stretch of the *vastus medialis*, and the second part emphasizes the stretch of the *vastus lateralis*. Be sure to stretch both legs. This stretch is most effective when done in a warm swimming pool, holding onto the edge for balance.

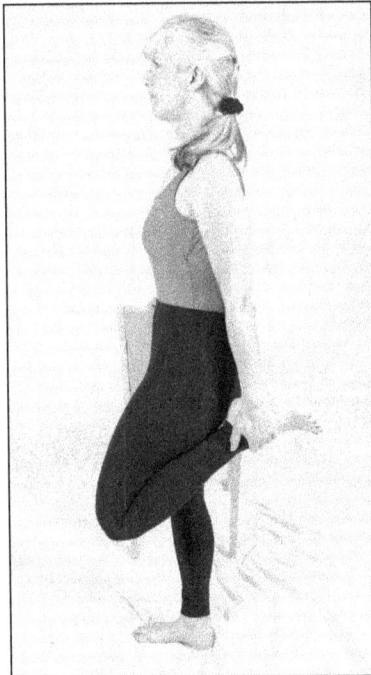

Thigh on same side   *Thigh on opposite side*

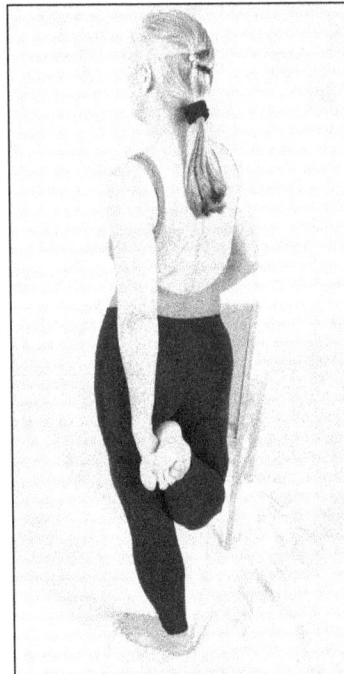

Also See:

* Hamstrings (chapter 8)
* Sartorius (chapter 7)
* Gluteus minimus (anterior portion, chapter 4)
* Adductor muscles of the hip (chapter 6)
* Soleus (chapter 11)
* Peroneus longus (chapter 13)

You may also need to search for trigger points in the *iliopsoas, tensor fasciae latae,* and *gluteus medius,* since trigger points in those muscles can either cause similar pain referral patterns or may be affected by *quadriceps femoris* muscle group trigger points in some way.

Since trigger points in these muscles don't directly cause knee, lower leg, ankle and foot pain, they are not addressed in this book. If you can't relieve your pain with the self-help techniques in this book after six to eight weeks, you may wish to consider whether you need to treat trigger points in these additional muscles, or if you still have perpetuating factors to resolve. Go to the end of this book for other books by the author that provide self-treatment techniques of muscles not covered in this book.

> **Differential Diagnosis:** There are many causes of knee pain, including ligament strains and tears, torn meniscuses, tendonitis, bursitis, kneecap fractures, and nerve entrapments. If you still have pain after inactivating trigger points, you will need to see an orthopedic doctor for evaluation. Even if other causes are found, there are also likely trigger points involved, and treatment can help prepare you for surgery and with recovery afterward.

Chapter 6: Adductor Muscles of the Hip

(Adductor Longus, Adductor Brevis, Adductor Magnus, and Gracilis)

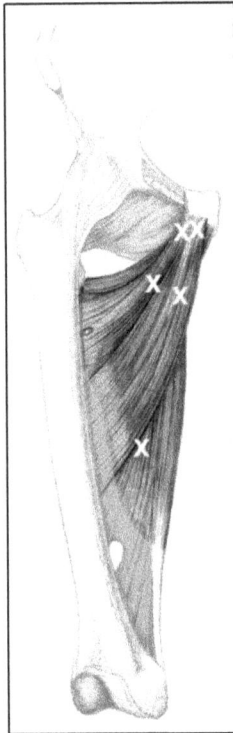

Front view of thigh --
Adductor muscles

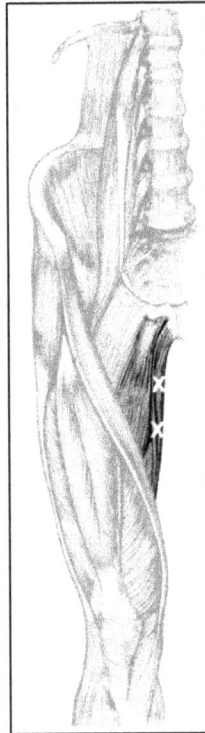

Front view of thigh --
Gracilis

Common Symptoms

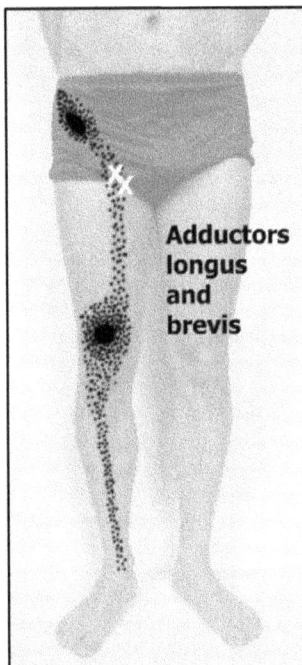

Adductors longus and brevis

Adductor Longus and Adductor Brevis
- referred pain on the front of your thigh, over the front of your knee, and down the inside of your lower leg
- pain feels deep
- trigger points may cause stiffness of your knee
- possibly pain may only be felt during vigorous activity or muscle overload
- pain is increased by standing and by sudden twists of your hip
- restricted range-of-motion in moving your thigh away from the midline of your body
- possibly restricted range-of-motion in rotating your thigh outward

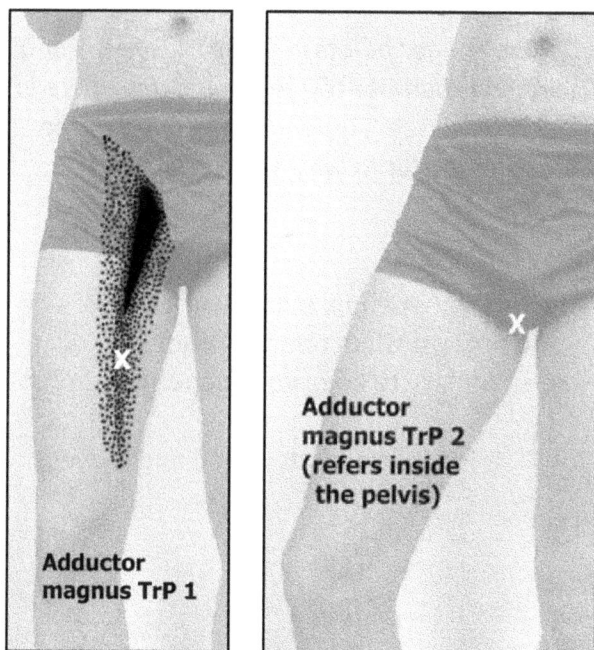

Adductor Magnus

- pain on the front-inside of your thigh, from your groin area down to the inside of your knee
- pain feels deep, possibly like it's shooting up into your pelvis and exploding like a firecracker
- the common trigger point high up between the legs may refer pain to your pubic bone, vagina, rectum, or possibly your bladder
- pain may only occur during intercourse
- difficulty getting comfortable at night

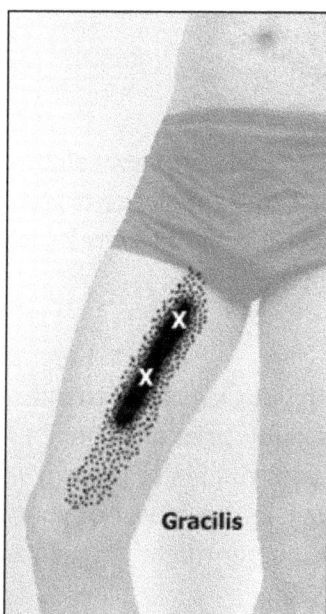

Adductor magnus TrP 2 (refers inside the pelvis)

Adductor magnus TrP 1

Gracilis

- pain on the inside of your thigh that feels hot, stingy, and superficial
- pain may be constant at rest, and no change of position relieves it except for walking

Gracilis

Causes and Perpetuation of Trigger Points

- a sudden overload, for example, trying to stop yourself from slipping on ice by trying to keep your legs from spreading
- horseback riding
- long bike trips (if you haven't trained for it)
- running up or down hills
- sitting for long periods, especially when driving, or with one leg crossed over the other knee
- skiing (most likely by snowplowing/wedge turns, or unexpectedly doing the "splits")

This is a list of perpetuating factors specific only to trigger points in <u>these</u> muscles. For a full list of perpetuating factors that can cause and perpetuate trigger points anywhere in the body and which also apply to these muscles, please see "Appendix A" (found at the end of this book), since some may need to be addressed for lasting pain relief.

Helpful Hints

- Be sure to read the section on perpetuating factors in Appendix A, particularly the sections on infections, nutritional problems, and organ dysfunction and disease.
- When sleeping, put a pillow between your knees, and try to keep your upper leg almost straight.
- Don't sit with your legs crossed, and if you must sit for long periods, stand and move around frequently.

Self-Help Techniques

Apply moist heat to the upper front and inner thigh.

Applying Pressure

Parts of these muscles are more difficult to treat on yourself, so you will probably also need the help of a massage therapist, acupuncturist, or physical therapist to treat all the trigger points. Since the *adductors magnus* and *brevis* trigger points are so deep, it is hard to work on these muscles with massage alone. Ultrasound is an effective treatment.

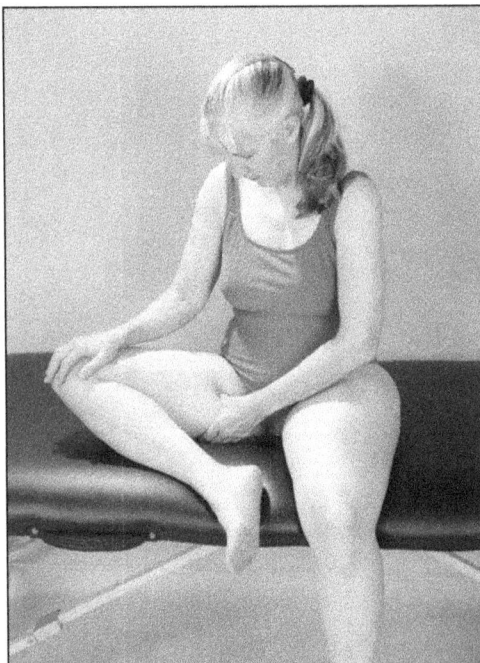

Hip Adductor Pressure: Sit with your legs bent to one side, with one heel close to the pubic area and the other one out to the side. Use your fingers or press a golf ball (or other pressure device in the center of your palm) into tender points on your inner thigh.

To access the upper portion of the *adductor magnus*, reach between your legs and find your sit bone with your fingers. Press the muscle attachment all around that area—it is easiest to use the hand of the opposite side. In addition to applying pressure to the *adductor* muscles, you may be able to lift and pinch part of this muscle group between the thumb and fingers of your opposite hand.

Stretches

Hip Adductor Stretch: Hold onto a chair back, spread your legs apart almost as far as you can with your toes pointed straight forward, and gently rotate your pelvis away from the side you are stretching.

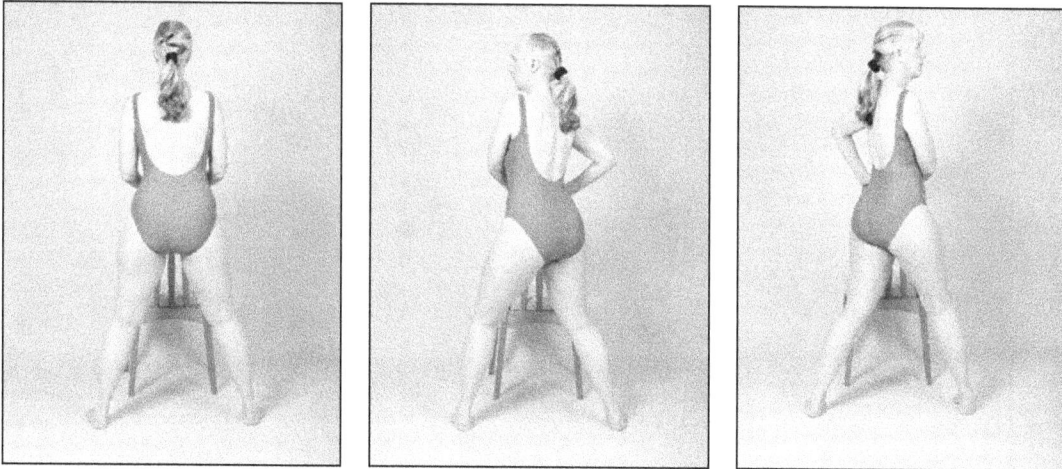

Pool Adductor Stretch: Hold onto a chair back, spread your legs apart almost as far as you can, and shift your weight to one side, allowing that knee to bend. The stretch is felt on the opposite inner thigh. It may be easier on your knees to do this stretch in a warm swimming pool in chest-deep water.

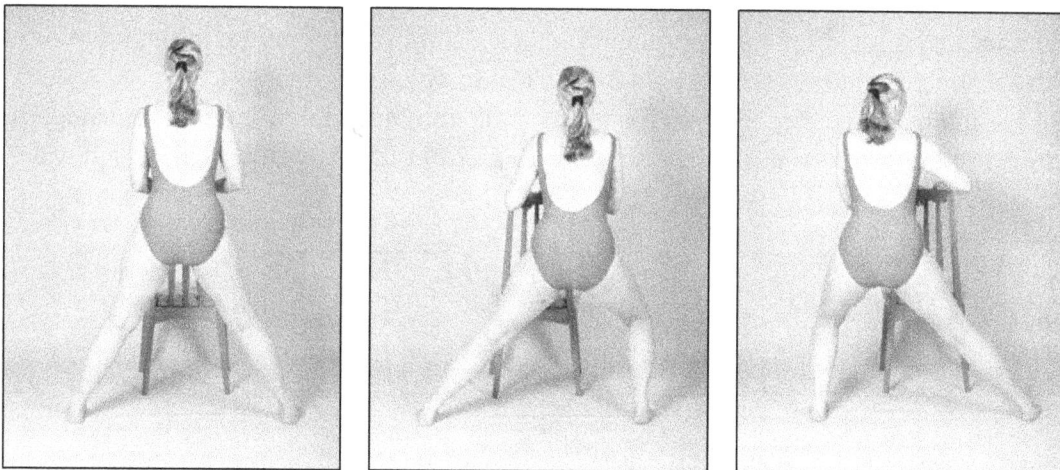

Also See:
* Vastus lateralis (chapter 5)

Differential Diagnosis: Three conditions may overload the hip *adductors* and cause chronic problems: pubic stress symphysitis, pubic stress fracture, and adductor insertion avulsion syndrome. If you are not able to relieve trigger points more than temporarily, you should see a health care provider to check for these conditions.

Chapter 7: Sartorius

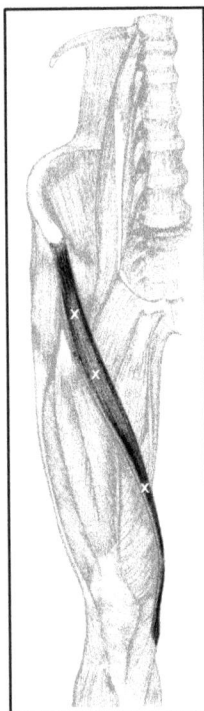

Front view of thigh

Common Symptoms

- referred pain that is superficial, sharp and tingling, felt at various points in the front of your thigh and possibly superficial pain on the inside of your knee
- if the lateral femoral cutaneous nerve is entrapped, you may feel numbness, burning, or uncomfortable sensations in the front of your thigh (meralgia paresthetica), which will be increased by standing or walking

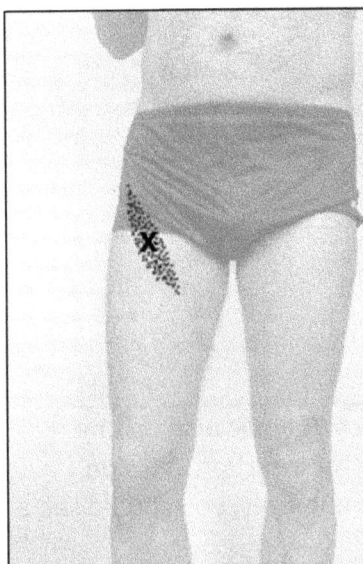

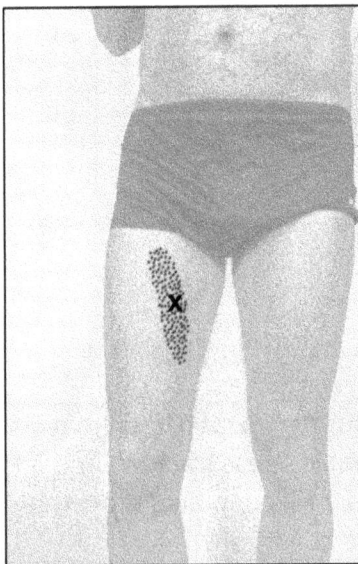

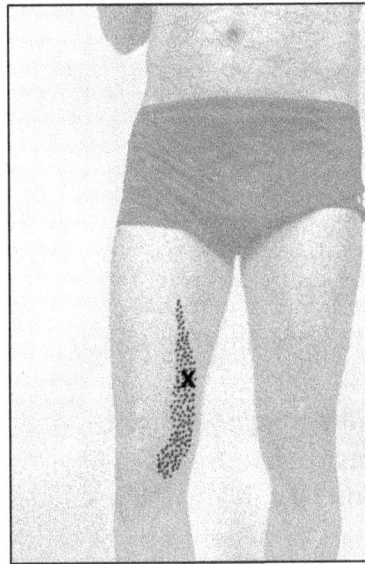

Causes and Perpetuation of Trigger Points

- excessive foot pronation
- possibly a twisting fall
- trigger points are usually found in conjunction with trigger points in the quadriceps femoris (*rectus femoris* and *vastus medialis*, chapter 5), *adductor* muscles of the hip (chapter 6), *iliopsoas*, *pectineus*, and *tensor fasciae latae*.

This is a list of perpetuating factors specific only to trigger points in <u>this</u> *muscle. For a full list of perpetuating factors that can cause and perpetuate trigger points anywhere in the body and which also apply to this muscle, please see "Appendix A" (found at the end of this book), since some may need to be addressed for lasting pain relief.*

Helpful Hints

- Trigger points in the lower part of the *sartorius* muscle refer pain in an area similar to the *vastus medialis*, but pain from *vastus medialis* trigger points will feel deep in the knee joint, rather than diffuse and superficial.
- If you have burning pain or odd sensations on the front of your thigh, try searching for trigger points below the pointy bony part of the front of your pelvis, and also work on the *iliopsoas*. "Meralgia paresthetica" (see above in "Common Symptoms") may be caused by obesity, constricting garments or belts, one leg anatomically shorter than the other, or carrying a wallet in the front pants pocket. These causes will need to be addressed in order to obtain lasting relief.
- Don't sit cross-legged in the lotus position, or with your ankle crossed over your opposite knee.
- Don't sleep with your knees drawn up tightly toward your chest. Place a pillow between your legs.

Self-Help Techniques

Be sure to search for trigger points in the quadriceps femoris (*rectus femoris* and *vastus medialis,* chapter 5), *adductor* muscles of the hip (chapter 6), *iliopsoas*, *pectineus*, and *tensor fasciae latae*, since the *sartorius* rarely develops trigger points on its own.

Applying Pressure

Sartorius Pressure: You may use the same pressure techniques as the *vastus medialis* and *rectus femoris* muscles (chapter 5), and you may also massage the muscle. Note how the muscle goes from the pointy part of the hip bone in front, crosses the front of the thigh, and then curves into your inner thigh as it approaches the knee. Be sure to work on all those areas so you won't miss the muscle.

Also See:

*   Rectus femoris and vastus medialis (chapter 5)
*   Adductor muscles of the hip (chapter 6)

You may also need to search for trigger points in the *iliopsoas*, *tensor fasciae latae*, and *pectineus* muscles, since trigger points in these muscles can affect or be affected by *sartorius* trigger points.

Since trigger points in these muscles don't directly cause knee, lower leg, ankle and foot pain, they are not addressed in this book. If you can't relieve your pain with the self-help techniques in this book after six to eight weeks, you may wish to consider whether you need to treat trigger points in these additional muscles, or if you still have perpetuating factors to resolve. Go to the end of this book for other books by the author that provide self-treatment techniques of muscles not covered in this book.

Chapter 8: Hamstrings

(Biceps Femoris, Semitendinosus, and Semimembranosus)

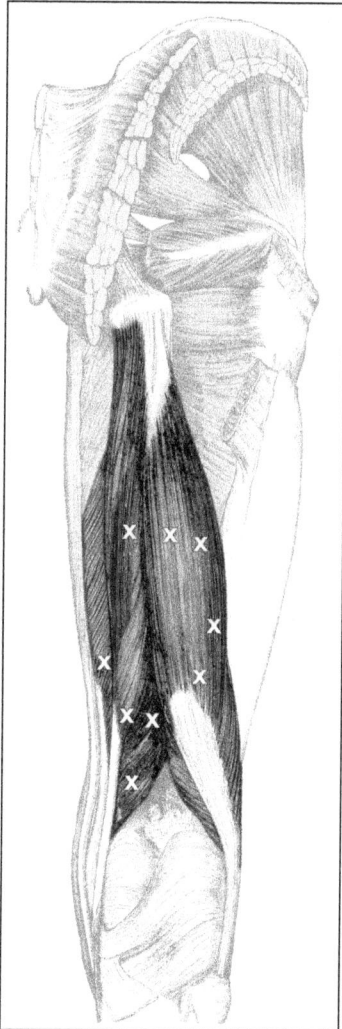

Referred pain from trigger points in the *hamstring* muscles frequently gets diagnosed by both patients and practitioners as "sciatic pain," because of the distribution pattern down the back of the leg. At least 80% of pain down the leg comes from trigger point referral, not from "pinched nerves," a herniated disc, or stenosis in a lumbar vertebra. Since "sciatica" is usually assumed to be caused by compression on a nerve, pain referrals from trigger points are probably more aptly called "pseudo-sciatica."

Back view, gluteal area and thigh

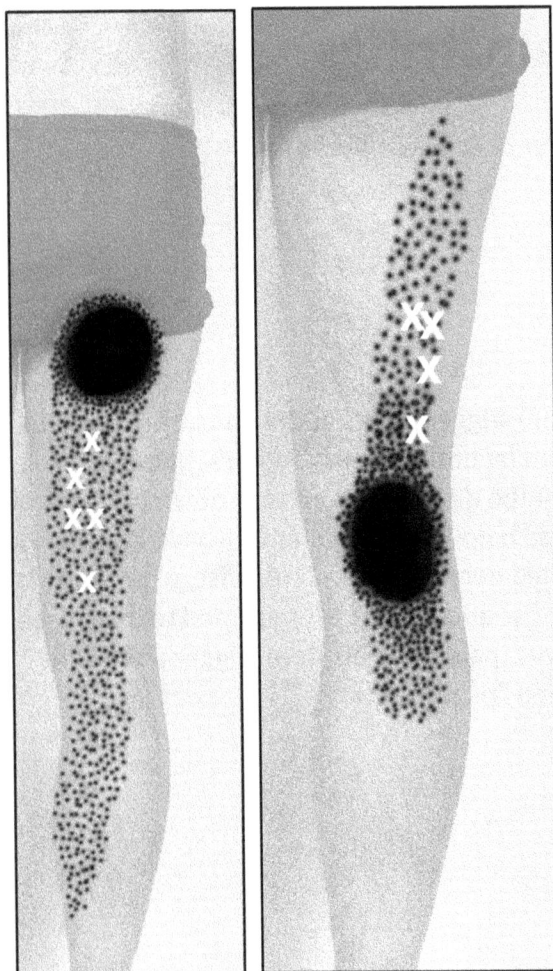

Common Symptoms

- referred pain over the back of the thigh, around the crease of the butt, over the back of the knee, and sometimes over the calf
- pain with walking, possibly even causing a limp
- pain with getting up from a chair, particularly if your legs have been crossed
- pain on the back of the thigh, knee, and crease area of the butt when sitting, due to pressure on the trigger points
- pain in the *biceps femoris* can disrupt sleep
- it may feel like the pain is only in the *quadriceps femoris* muscle (chapter 5, the front of the thigh) when in fact the problem is originating in the *hamstrings*, and causing trigger points to form in the *quadriceps femoris* group
- tingling and numbness when sitting in a chair that is too high
- restricted range-of-motion when bending forward to reach your toes
- in above-knee amputees, phantom limb pain may come from trigger points in the *hamstrings*, particularly if the muscle was stretched to cover the bone

Causes and Perpetuation of Trigger Points

- strain or partial tears of the *hamstrings* as a result of inadequate stretching before a sports activity
- sitting in a chair where your feet don't touch the ground (more common in shorter people)
- sitting on a ski lift without a footrest
- children sitting in a high chair without a footrest
- a small hemipelvis (either the right or left half of the pelvis)
- treatment of *quadriceps femoris* trigger points without also treating the *hamstrings*
- auto accidents regardless of the direction of impact (in about 25% of accidents)
- short upper arms in relation to torso height that cause you to shift your weight forward when sitting

This is a list of perpetuating factors specific only to trigger points in these muscles. For a full list of perpetuating factors that can cause and perpetuate trigger points anywhere in the body and which also apply to these muscles, please see "Appendix A" (found at the end of this book), since some may need to be addressed for lasting pain relief.

Helpful Hints

- If your chair is too high for you (you should be able to easily slip your fingers between your chair and thigh), buy or build a sloped footstool. Patio chairs can cause problems if there is a metal bar across the front and a sagging seat bottom.
- Make sure children in high-chairs have footrests, and those at school have chairs or footrests of the proper height.
- If you swim, don't use the crawl stroke too much, but instead vary it with other strokes.
- If you bicycle, be sure your seat height is high enough that your legs can straighten out as much as possible without your knees locking.
- When driving for long periods, use cruise-control and take frequent breaks.
- You may get mis-diagnosed with sciatica, since the pain from sciatica is similar to that of *hamstrings* trigger points.
- If you have pain remaining after a laminectomy, check the *hamstrings* for trigger points.

Self-Help Techniques

Caution: *Do not apply pressure to your legs if you have varicose veins in the area to be treated—it could release a clot that could go to your heart or brain! An acupuncturist or massage therapist should treat your legs, because they can avoid varicose veins.* However, you may still do the stretches and exercises below.

You may need to treat the *gluteus minimus* (chapter 4), *paraspinals*, *gluteus maximus*, *gluteus medius*, and/or *piriformis* first, since these muscles can restrict range of motion, can have similar referral patterns, and/or keep *hamstrings* trigger points activated.

Applying Pressure

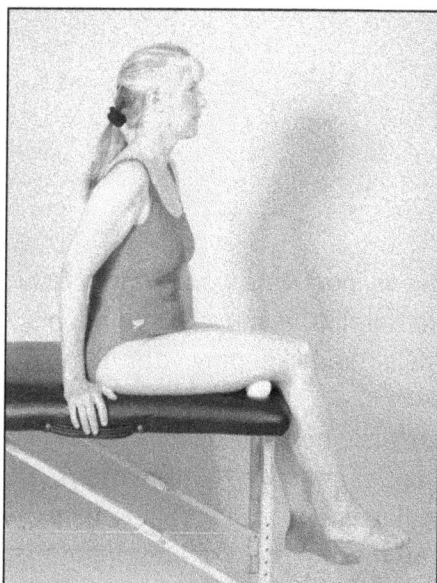

Hamstrings Pressure: Sit on a surface where your legs can dangle but are fully supported along the length of the thigh. Place a tennis ball under one thigh and use your hand to move the ball around to treat tender points. Repeat on the opposite thigh.

You may also treat the inner-thigh *hamstrings* by using your opposite hand to pinch the muscles between your thumb and fingers.

Stretches

In-Bathtub Stretch: With your head hanging forward, lean forward and reach your hands down toward your toes, until you are feeling a gentle stretch. Relax and then repeat, moving your hands further down each time, but only as far down as you can feel a gentle stretch. Do this in a hot bath if you can. [**Note**: If you have trigger points in the *iliopsoas* muscle, even if they aren't active trigger points, this stretch can cause a reactive cramp.]

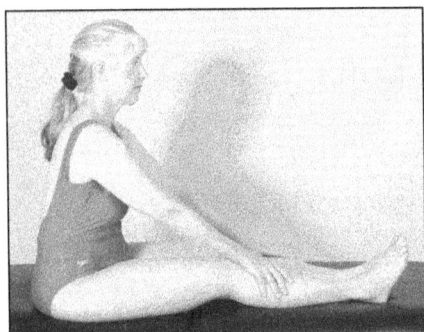

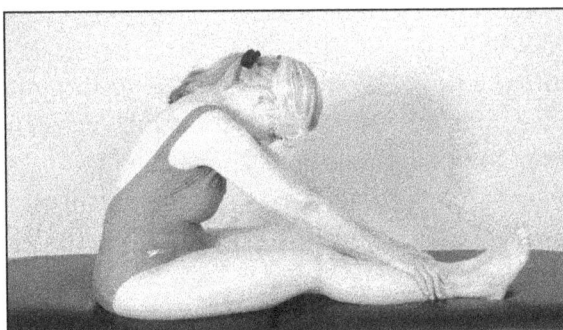

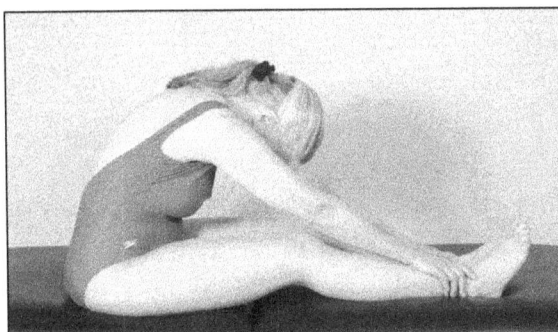

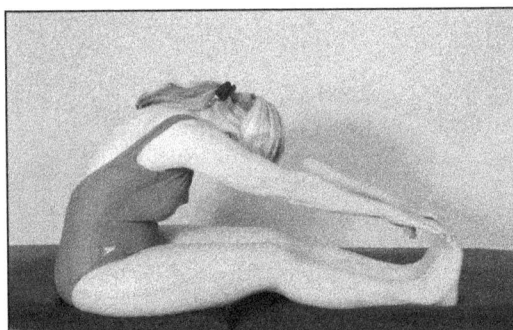

Also See:
* Gluteus minimus (posterior portion, chapter 4)
* Popliteus (chapter 9)
* Gastrocnemius (chapter 10)
* Vastus lateralis (chapter 5)
* Adductor magnus (chapter 6)
* Plantaris (chapter 11)

You may need to condition the *gluteus maximus* in order to inactivate *hamstring* trigger points. To condition the *gluteus maximus*, you must swim, hike uphill (this muscle is minimally used for normal walking), jump, or do some other vigorous activity while keeping your heart rate within your optimal range for aerobic respiration.

You may also need to search for trigger points in the *posterior neck, pectoralis minor, infraspinatus, subscapularis, teres minor,* and *supraspinatus* muscles, since tight *hamstrings* also affect these muscles. Tight *hamstrings* will tend to cause a flattened lumbar spine and a head-forward posture, resulting in problems in the *quadratus lumborum, paraspinals, iliopsoas,* and *rectus abdominis* muscles. You should check these muscles for trigger points, particularly if you have upper-body symptoms that are only temporarily relieved.

You may also need to search for trigger points in the *piriformis, obturator internus, gluteus medius,* and *iliopsoas,* since trigger points in those muscles can either cause similar pain referral patterns or may affect or be affected by *hamstrings* trigger points in some way.

Since trigger points in these muscles don't directly cause knee, lower leg, ankle and foot pain, they are not addressed in this book. If you can't relieve your pain with the self-help techniques in this book after six to eight weeks, you may wish to consider whether you need to treat trigger points in these additional muscles, or if you still have perpetuating factors to resolve. Go to the end of this book for other books by the author that provide self-treatment techniques of muscles not covered in this book.

> **Differential Diagnosis:** If you are unable to relieve your symptoms with trigger point self-help techniques, you may need to see a health care provider to rule out osteoarthritis of the knee. Misalignment of the sacroiliac joint and L_4 to L_5 and L_5 to S_1 vertebrae can cause spasm and restriction of the *hamstring* muscles. See a chiropractor or osteopathic physician for evaluation and treatment.

Chapter 9: Popliteus

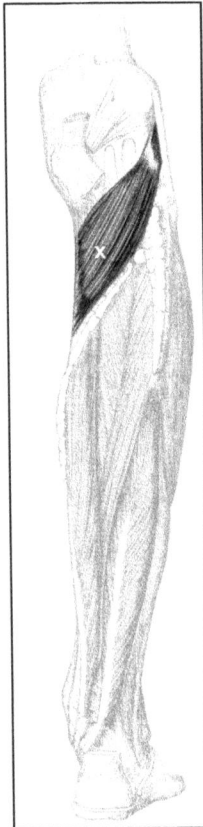

Back of leg

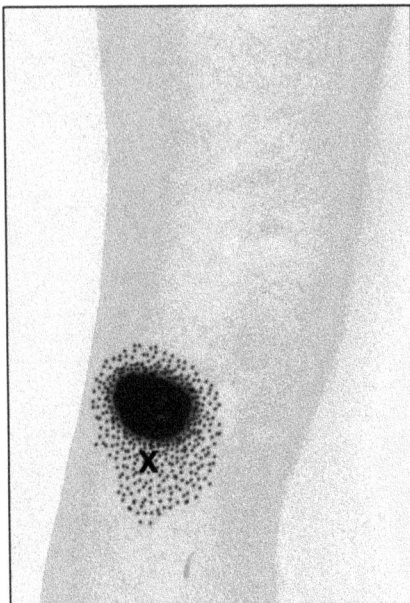

Back of knee

Common Symptoms

- pain referred to the back of your knee when crouching, running, or walking
- pain is worse when going downstairs or downhill
- a slight decrease in range-of-motion, which may likely be unnoticeable
- trigger points are usually found after trigger points in the *gastrocnemius* (chapter 10) or *biceps femoris* (chapter 8) have been inactivated
- knee pain with straightening your leg

Causes and Perpetuation of Trigger Points

- sports that require you to twist, slide, and change direction suddenly, such as soccer, football, and baseball
- running or skiing downhill
- a trauma or strain that tears the posterior cruciate ligament in the knee
- foot pronation, especially combined with the above activities
- trigger points can develop in conjunction with a tear of the *plantaris* muscle

This is a list of perpetuating factors specific only to trigger points in <u>this</u> muscle. For a full list of perpetuating factors that can cause and perpetuate trigger points anywhere in the body and which also apply to this muscle, please see "Appendix A" (found at the end of this book), since some may need to be addressed for lasting pain relief.

Helpful Hints

- If you do any of the above sports activities, you may need to condition this muscle gradually, with the help of a physical therapist.
- Gradually add distance to your runs or hikes, rather than suddenly increasing the mileage.
- Prior to an aggravating activity, take extra vitamin C, and be sure to keep your legs warm.
- Avoid running or walking on side-slanted surfaces, or at least change directions periodically so you are running on the opposite slant (i.e., return on the same side of the road, instead of crossing and always facing traffic).
- Do not wear high heels.
- Get corrective orthotics to correct foot pronation problems.

Self-Help Techniques

Applying Pressure

Do not apply pressure to your legs if you have varicose veins in the area to be treated -- it could release a clot that could go to your heart or brain! *An acupuncturist or massage therapist should treat your legs, because they can avoid the veins.* You may still do the stretches and exercises below.

Gastrocnemius Pressure: Do the *gastrocnemius* self-work first, being careful to work close to the back crease of the knee. See chapter 10.

Popliteus Pressure: Sit in a chair and bend forward slightly, supporting yourself with one hand on a thigh. To work on the part of the muscle closest to the outside of your knee, use the hand on the same side. To work on the part of the muscle closest to the inside of your knee, use your thumb of the opposite hand; the bulk of the muscle is on the inside. If you keep your thumb straight, it is easier to press through the overlaying muscles into the trigger points in the *popliteus*. Be sure to get close to the crease of the knee to treat the entire muscle, but *don't press right into the crease behind the knee -- there are veins and nerves that are close to the surface.* You may need the help of a massage therapist.

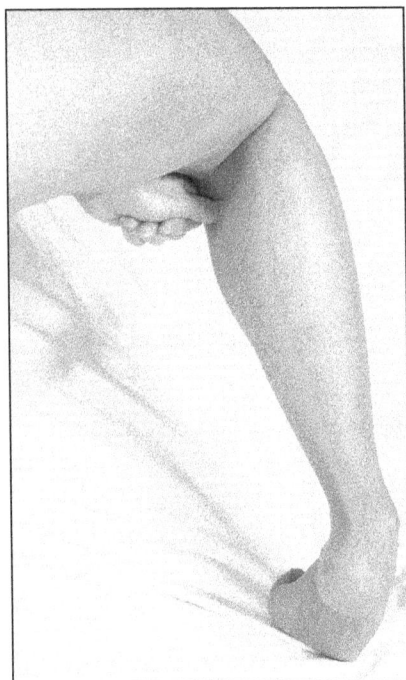

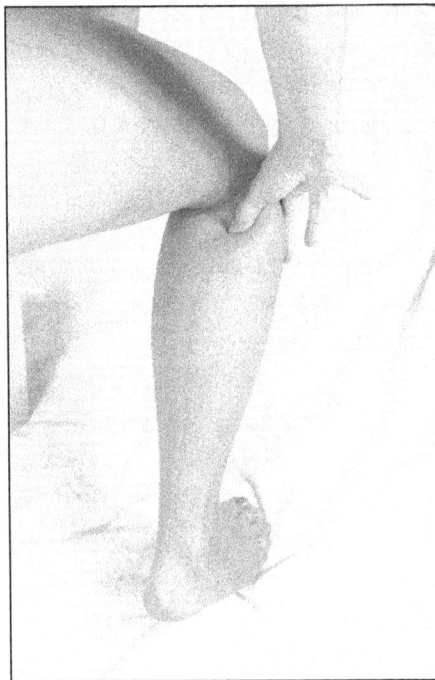

Also See:
*   Gastrocnemius (chapter 10)
*   Biceps femoris (chapter 8)

Differential Diagnosis: If you are unable to relieve your symptoms with trigger point self-help techniques, you may need to see a health care provider to rule out a Baker's cyst, thrombosis of the popliteal vein, anteromedial and posterolateral instability of the knee, avulsion of the popliteus tendon, or a meniscus tear.

Chapter 10: Gastrocnemius

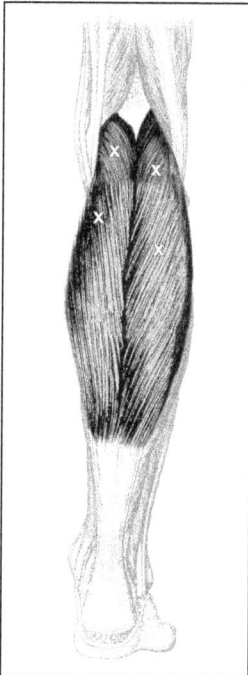

The Achilles tendon attaches the *gastrocnemius* and *soleus* muscles to the heel bone. If the tendon feels tight, work on the muscle bellies to relax the tendon.

Rear view of leg

Common Symptoms

- pain referred into the arch of your foot, over the back of your leg and knee, and possibly the back of your lower thigh
- pain with climbing steep slopes, over rocks, or walking on slanted surfaces
- calf cramps when sleeping
- difficulty walking fast, and a tendency to walk with a flat-footed, stiff-legged gait
- difficulty straightening your leg completely when standing

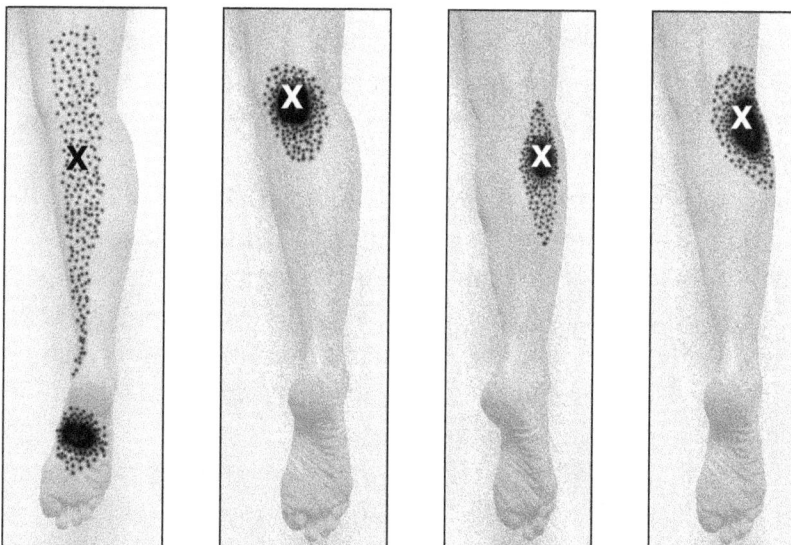

Causes and Perpetuation of Trigger Points

- muscle chilling
- prolonged immobility with your toes pointed, such as when sleeping
- impaired circulation
- walking, climbing, or running up steep slopes, over rocks, or on slanted surfaces
- riding a bicycle with the seat too low
- standing while leaning forward for a prolonged time
- wearing a cast
- wearing socks, garters, or knee-high hose with an elastic band that is too tight
- wearing high heels
- hooking your heel on a rung of a stool for a prolonged time
- driving a car with an accelerator pedal that is too horizontal
- sitting in a chair with a high front edge that impairs circulation or otherwise compresses the backs of your thighs
- sitting in a reclining chair that places a lot of your leg weight on your calves
- viral infections
- jobs that require a lot of squatting, such as mechanics

This is a list of perpetuating factors specific only to trigger points in <u>this</u> muscle. For a full list of perpetuating factors that can cause and perpetuate trigger points anywhere in the body and which also apply to this muscle, please see "Appendix A" (found at the end of this book), since some may need to be addressed for lasting pain relief.

Helpful Hints

- Calf cramps are one of the most common symptoms of *gastrocnemius* trigger points, and often occur when sleeping or sitting for too long with the toes pointed. If this happens, rather than standing and walking immediately, instead gently flex your foot so your toes are moving toward your trunk, and then release.
- To reduce the tendency for your calves to cramp when sleeping, keep them warm at night by using a heating pad at bedtime, or use an electric blanket. Sleep with a warm covering on your legs, such as knee-high pile socks or long-johns. During the day, keep your calves and body warm. Use a space heater near your legs if necessary.
- At night, place a pillow against the bottom of your feet to maintain a 90-degree angle between your feet and lower leg.
- Calf cramps may be brought on by dehydration, loss of/or inadequate intake of electrolytes (including potassium, calcium, magnesium, and salt), hypoparathyroidism, Parkinson's disease, and possibly diabetes. If you are experiencing calf cramps, try increasing your water intake and take a multi-mineral supplement. If you limit your salt intake severely and/or sweat heavily, try increasing your salt intake, unless otherwise directed by a health care provider. Some drugs can cause calf cramps, such as lithium, cimetidine, bumetanide, vincristine, and phenothiazines.
- Dr.'s Travell and Simons found that taking vitamin-E (400 I.U. per day) helped some patients tremendously. If you take a multi-vitamin be sure to count that amount of vitamin-E toward the 400 I.U., and only take the larger dose for a maximum of two

weeks, or less if the cramps disappear sooner. Try vitamin B-2 (riboflavin) if you have calf cramps during pregnancy.

- Don't wear high heels, and avoid hooking your heels on the rung of a stool. Avoid wearing smooth leather shoes, particularly on a slippery floor.
- Use a car with an accelerator pedal that isn't too stiff. If the accelerator pedal in your car is at a steep vertical angle, try putting a wedge on the pedal with the big end at the bottom to reduce the angle of your foot. If it is nearly horizontal, try putting the big end of the wedge at the top. Using cruise control will help. Take breaks every 30-60 minutes.
- Sit in a chair at the proper height for you so it isn't restricting circulation in the back of your thighs, and use a slanted footstool to elevate your lower legs if necessary. Using a rocking chair prevents prolonged immobility and increases circulation.
- If you swim, avoid the crawl stroke, since the kick causes you to point your toes.
- If your socks or hose leave a mark or indentation on your skin at the elastic band, the elastic is too tight and is cutting off needed circulation. Buy socks and hose with a wider, looser band.
- Until the trigger points are inactivated, avoid walking up hills or on slanted surfaces.
- Stretch before and after athletic activities.
- "Posterior compartment syndrome" is where increased pressure within the muscle compartment adversely affects blood and lymph circulation of the muscles inside. The superficial posterior compartment contains the *soleus* (chapter 11) and *gastrocnemius* muscles. See the discussion on "Compartment Syndrome" in chapter 1; it is important to see a doctor *immediately* if you have this condition. Once successfully treated, you should subsequently check for trigger points, since they were likely formed as a result of posterior compartment syndrome.
- If you have had a laminectomy in the lumbar area and still experience pain in the back of the leg, try searching for trigger points.

Self-Help Techniques

Check the *gluteus minimus* (posterior portion, chapter 4) to ascertain whether trigger points there are causing and perpetuating satellite trigger points in the *gastrocnemius*. Also, check the *tibialis anterior* (chapter 14) and *long extensors* of toes (chapter 16) for associated trigger points.

If the Achilles' tendon feels tight, work on the *gastrocnemius* and *soleus* (chapter 11) muscle bellies to relax the tendon.

Applying Pressure

Do not apply pressure to your legs if you have varicose veins in the area to be treated -- it could release a clot that could go to your heart or brain! *An acupuncturist or massage therapist should treat your legs, because they can avoid the veins.* You may still do the stretches and exercises below.

Gastrocnemius Pressure: Lay face-up with your butt scooted up close to a chair, coffee table, or other hard surface that is about the height you need to get a 90° angle bend at your knee. Place the ball on the hard surface and rest your calf on it, with gravity giving you the needed pressure. Be sure to work as much as you can top to bottom, and rotate your leg side to side to get as much of the edges of the muscles as you can. You can move your leg over the ball; be sure to hold each point eight seconds to one minute, following the general guidelines. You will need to move the ball with your at least hand once to get all the points.

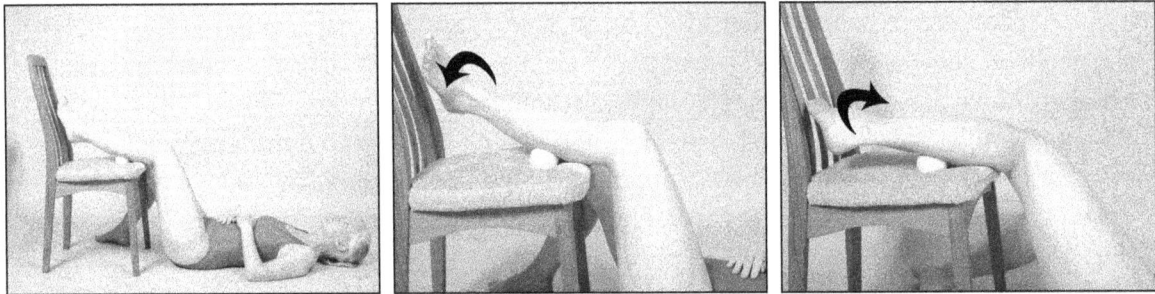

Then, sit up with your legs bent to one side, with one heel close to the pubic area and the other one out to the side. Holding a golf ball, tennis ball, or some other pressure device in the center of your palm, press the device into tender points on your inner and outer lower legs to work the edges of the muscles.

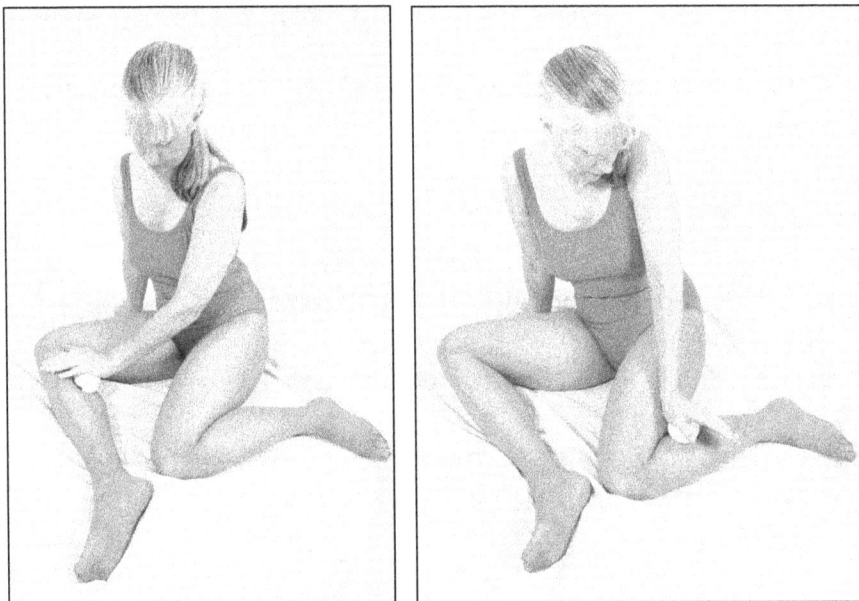

Stretches

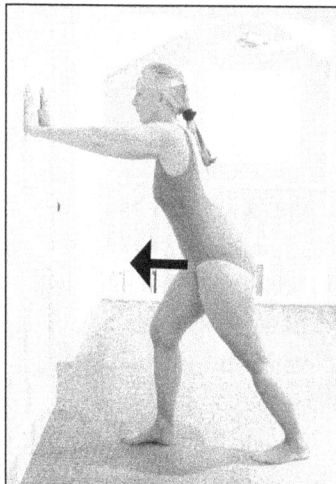

Gastrocnemius Stretch: Stand a short distance from a wall, and place your hands on the wall at about head height. Place the leg to be stretched out behind you, with your knee straight, your heel on the floor, and your toes pointing straight forward. Let your hips move forward until you are getting a gentle stretch on the back of your lower leg. Look straight ahead so your neck is not bent down.

Seated Gastrocnemius Stretch: Sit with your back against a wall with your legs out straight, and put a thin, long towel around one foot and hold both ends with your hands. Gently press the ball of your foot against the towel for five seconds, while you slowly inhale. As you exhale, release the pressure on your foot and use the towel to pull the ball of the foot toward you, giving you a gentle stretch on the back of the calf. Repeat three or four times with each foot.

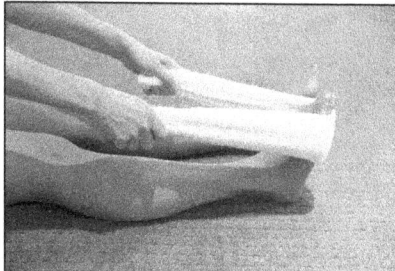

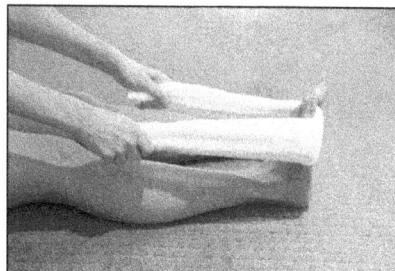

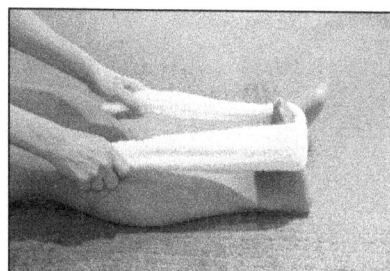

Also See:
* Soleus (chapter 11)
* Hamstrings (chapter 8)
* Gluteus minimus (posterior portion, chapter 4)
* Tibialis anterior (chapter 14)
* Long extensors of toes (chapter 16)

Differential Diagnosis: If the self-help techniques do not relieve the trigger points more than temporarily, you may need to see a health care provider to rule out damage to the nerve roots at the S_1 level. You may also need to rule out a partial tear in the muscle ("tennis leg"), posterior compartment syndrome, thrombophlebitis, intermittent claudication, arteriosclerosis, or Baker's cyst.

Chapter 11: Soleus

(Soleus, Plantaris)

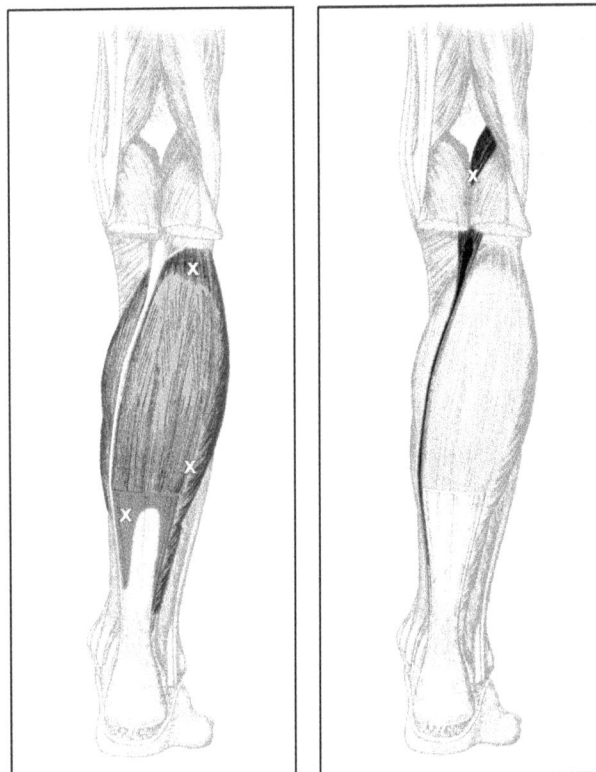

The *soleus* muscle is known as the body's "second heart," due to its pumping action that returns blood from the lower leg to the heart. Flexing and extending the foot can greatly improve circulation in the legs.

Views of back of leg

Soleus   **Plantaris**

Common Symptoms

- trigger points cause an inability to flex the foot toward your knee, making it difficult to squat or kneel down to pick items up off the floor, which can subsequently lead to back pain due to improper lifting
- difficulty walking due to pain, especially uphill and up or down stairs

Soleus
- the most common trigger point in the *soleus* refers pain to the back and bottom of the heel, and the Achilles tendon
- the second most common trigger point in the *soleus* is located close to the back of your knee and refers pain to the upper half of the back of your calf
- an uncommon trigger point refers pain over the sacroiliac joint on the same side
- *soleus* trigger points may be the cause of "growing pains" in children
- trigger points and subsequent tightness of the *soleus* can entrap the posterior tibial veins, posterior tibial artery, and tibial nerve, causing swelling of your foot and ankle and severe heel pain and tingling

Plantaris

- trigger points in the *plantaris* muscle refer pain behind your knee and to the upper half of your calf
- the *plantaris* can entrap the popliteal artery, which can cause calf pain

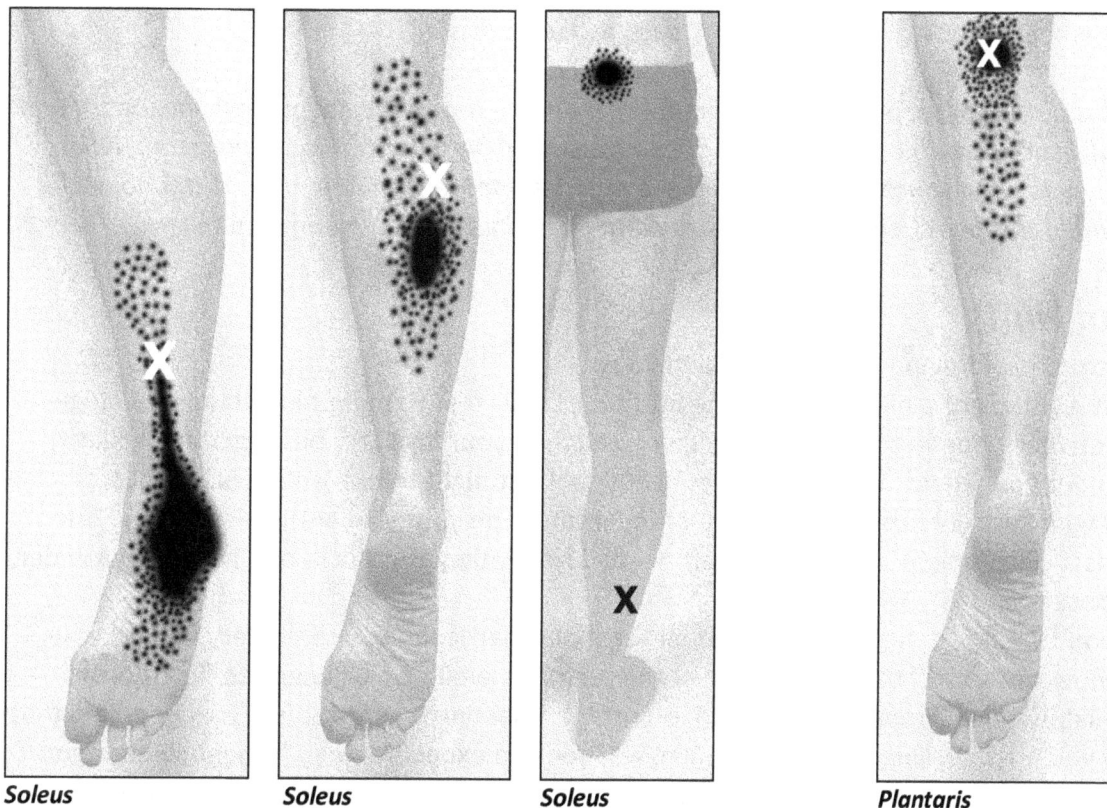

Soleus   *Soleus*   *Soleus*   *Plantaris*

Causes and Perpetuation of Trigger Points

- running / jogging
- a direct blow to the muscle
- a fall or near-fall
- referral from trigger points in the *gluteus minimus* muscle (posterior portion, chapter 4)
- chilling of your calf, especially combined with immobility
- wearing smooth-soled shoes on slippery surfaces
- wearing high heels
- wearing shoes that are too stiff
- sitting in a chair that is too high, so that you are not able to keep your feet flat on the ground
- sitting in a chair with a high front edge that impairs circulation or otherwise compresses the back of your thighs
- sitting in a reclining chair that puts a lot of the leg weight on your calves
- prolonged immobility with your toes pointed, such as when sleeping
- wearing socks or knee-high hose with an elastic band that is too tight
- skiing or ice skating without stiff boots

- walking, climbing, or running up steep slopes, over rocks, or on slanted surfaces, especially when you are not used to it
- sustained pressure against your calf
- one leg anatomically shorter than the other, since the short side bears more of your body weight
- jobs that require a lot of squatting, such as mechanics

This is a list of perpetuating factors specific only to trigger points in <u>these</u> muscles. For a full list of perpetuating factors that can cause and perpetuate trigger points anywhere in the body and which also apply to these muscles, please see "Appendix A" (found at the end of this book), since some may need to be addressed for lasting pain relief.

Helpful Hints
- Stretch before and after athletic activities.
- At night, place a pillow against the bottom of your feet to maintain a 90-degree angle between your feet and lower leg. If you sleep on your back, try putting a small pillow under your knees. Wear knee-high fleece socks at night to prevent muscle chilling.
- If your socks or hose leave a mark or indentation on your skin at the elastic band, the elastic is too tight and is cutting off needed circulation. Buy socks and hose with a wider, looser band.
- Don't wear high heels or smooth leather shoes, particularly on a slippery floor. If your shoes are so stiff they don't bend at the toes very well, you will need to find more pliable shoes. Proper shoes are so important to lasting relief of *soleus* trigger points that if you are unwilling to change your shoes, you can expect to need frequent treatment.
- Sit in a chair at the proper height for you so it isn't restricting circulation in the back of your thighs, and use a slanted footstool to elevate your lower legs if necessary. Using a rocking chair prevents prolonged immobility and increases circulation. Most recliner chairs or footrests place too much pressure on the calf. If you choose to use some kind of lower leg support, make sure you get something that supports the whole back of your lower leg and heels so that no one area takes all the weight of the leg.
- When driving for long periods, take frequent breaks and use cruise control.
- Until the trigger points are inactivated, avoid walking up hills or on slanted surfaces.
- If you have pain with walking up stairs, try rotating your body to 45-degrees (instead of facing forward), keep your body erect, and put your entire foot on the next step, rather than letting your heel hang off of the edge.
- If you have one leg anatomically shorter than the other, you will need to see a specialist for compensating lifts.
- If you have heel pain and a bone spur is found on the bottom of the big bone of the heel, don't assume the spur is the source of the pain. The other heel may have a spur that causes no pain, so trigger points may be the source of the pain rather than the spur. An elevated serum uric acid level will cause a heel spur to become painful, and is likely to aggravate trigger points in the *soleus* and other muscles.
- Achilles tendinitis may be due to trigger points causing shortening of the *soleus* and *gastrocnemius* (chapter 10) muscles. Pain will be diffuse and possibly burning in or

around the Achilles tendon, and aggravated by activity. If the condition is severe, there also may be swelling, crackling sounds, or a tender nodule in the tendon. The cause is usually improper or over-training. Corrective orthotics and shoes with a more flexible sole may help considerably.

- The generic term "shin splints" has used in the past to refer to any chronic pain in the front or middle of the lower leg associated with exercise. More recently, "shin splints" refers specifically to irritation of the surface of the bone along the attachment of a muscle, and is called "periosteal irritation," or in the case of the *soleus*, "soleus periostalgia syndrome." This is caused by repetitive exercise, such as running or aerobic dancing. At first, pain will be mild and occur later in the exercise, and will be relieved by rest. As the condition progresses, pain will be more intense, occur earlier in the exercise, and may not be relieved once the exercise has stopped. The surface of the bone (periosteum) where the *soleus* attaches on the inside of the lower leg can be loosened and sometimes separated from the deeper part of the bone. A stress fracture can cause similar symptoms.
- "Posterior compartment syndrome" is where increased pressure within the muscle compartment adversely affects blood and lymph circulation of the muscles inside. The superficial posterior compartment contains the *soleus* and *gastrocnemius* (chapter 10) muscles. See the discussion on "Compartment Syndrome" in chapter 1; it is important to see a doctor *immediately* if you have this condition. Once successfully treated, you should subsequently check for trigger points, since they were likely formed as a result of posterior compartment syndrome.

Self-Help Techniques

Also check the *quadratus plantae* (chapter 18), since it can also cause pain on the bottom of the heel. If you have trigger points in the *soleus* and also have knee pain, search for trigger points in the *quadriceps femoris* (chapter 5), since loss of function in the calf puts additional stress on the front-of-the-thigh muscles.

If the Achilles' tendon feels tight, work on the *gastrocnemius* (chapter 10) and *soleus* muscle bellies to relax the tendon.

Applying Pressure

Do not apply pressure to your legs if you have varicose veins in the area to be treated -- it could release a clot that could go to your heart or brain! *An acupuncturist or massage therapist should treat your legs, because they can avoid the veins.* You may still do the stretches and exercises below.

Gastrocnemius Pressure: The *gastrocnemius* pressure will also treat the underlying *soleus* muscle. See chapter 10.

Stretches

Soleus Stretch: Hold onto something for support and place one foot out in front of you, and one foot slightly behind you, with the toes of both feet pointing straight forward. Keeping your heel on the floor, bend the knee of the rear foot until you are getting a gentle stretch in the *soleus* muscle. Look straight ahead so your neck is not bent down.

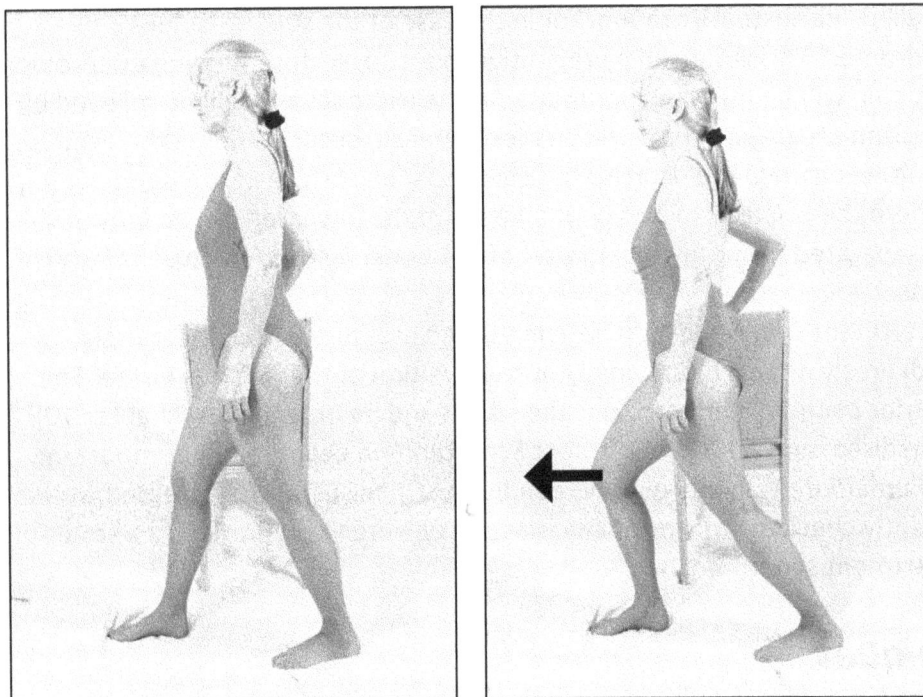

Also See:
* Quadratus plantae (chapter 18)
* Abductor hallucis (chapter 17)
* Gastrocnemius (chapter 10)
* Tibialis posterior (chapter 12)
* Long flexors of toes (chapter 15)
* Tibialis anterior (chapter 14)
* Extensor digitorum longus, extensor hallucis longus (chapter 16)
* Peroneus tertius (chapter 13)

Differential Diagnosis: If you are unable to relieve your symptoms with trigger point self-help techniques, you may need to see a health care provider to rule out a rupture of a calf muscle, S_1 nerve root irritation, thrombophlebitis, a ruptured popliteal cyst, or possibly a systemic viral infection. A ruptured muscle will cause sudden, intense pain at the time of an injury, followed by bruising that appears within one to two days. With thrombophlebitis there will be constant pain unaffected by activity level, and warmth and redness in the area.

Chapter 12: Tibialis Posterior

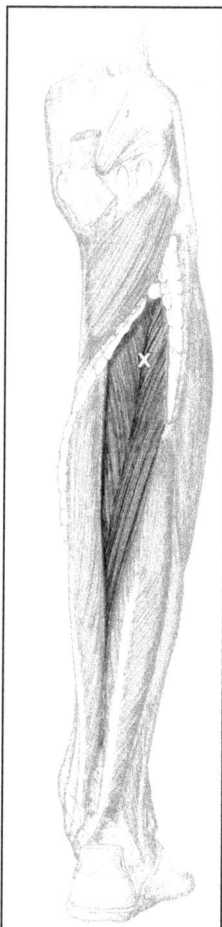

Common Symptoms

- referred pain primarily over the Achilles' tendon, with spillover pain through your heel, bottom of your foot and toes, and over the back of your calf
- pain in your foot when running or walking, especially on uneven surfaces

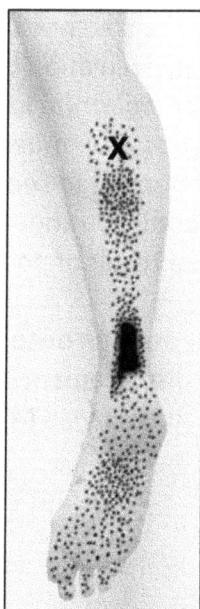

Back view of leg

Causes and Perpetuation of Trigger Points

- running or jogging, especially on uneven ground or side-slanted surfaces
- shoes that are worn down on the inside or outside edges
- foot pronation
- longer second toe (causing an unstable ankle and foot rocking)
- hyperuricemia with or without symptoms of gout in the big toe (diagnosed with a blood test)
- polymyalgia rheumatica (diagnosed with a blood test)

This is a list of perpetuating factors specific only to trigger points in <u>this</u> *muscle. For a full list of perpetuating factors that can cause and perpetuate trigger points anywhere in the body and which also apply to this muscle, please see "Appendix A" (found at the end of this book), since some may need to be addressed for lasting pain relief.*

Helpful Hints

- Get a good orthotic with arch support and a deep heel cup to prevent pronation.
- Avoid high heels and shoes that don't fit properly.
- Only walk or run on smooth, level surfaces until trigger points are inactivated. If you are unable to walk or run, try swimming and bicycling.
- See the discussion on "Shin Splints" in chapter 1. In the case of the *tibialis posterior*, shin splints usually develop in runners who are novices, or athletes who are poorly conditioned. At first, pain will be mild and occur later in the exercise, and will be relieved by rest. As the condition progresses, pain will be more intense, occur earlier in the exercise, and may not be relieved once the exercise has stopped. The surface of the bone (periosteum) where the *tibialis posterior* attaches on the tibia can be loosened and sometimes separated from the deeper part of the bone.
- "Posterior compartment syndrome" is where increased pressure within the muscle compartment adversely affects blood and lymph circulation of the muscles inside. The deep posterior compartment contains the *flexor digitorum longus*, *flexor hallucis longus* (chapter 15), *popliteus* (chapter 9), and *tibialis posterior* muscles. See the discussion on "Compartment Syndrome" in chapter 1; it is important to see a doctor *immediately* if you have this condition. Once successfully treated, you should subsequently check for trigger points, since they were likely formed as a result of posterior compartment syndrome.
- If a tight *posterior tibialis* is not treated, the tendon can become elongated, accompanied by severe pain with walking and displacement of the bones of the foot. The tendon can also rupture. This requires diagnosis by an MRI.

Self-Help Techniques

Applying Pressure

Do not apply pressure to your legs if you have varicose veins in the area to be treated -- it could release a clot that could go to your heart or brain! *An acupuncturist, physical therapist, or massage therapist should treat your legs, because they can avoid the veins.*

Gastrocnemius Pressure: The *gastrocnemius* pressure will help treat the *tibialis posterior*. See chapter 10. The *tibialis posterior* is deep and next to the bone, so you may not be able to get to the whole muscle with self-help techniques. It is difficult to inject this muscle and not recommended. Ultrasound and stretching are effective, so you may need to see a physical therapist or other professional that can help with this.

Also See:
* Flexor digitorum longus, flexor hallucis longus (chapter 15)
* Peroneus longus, peroneus brevis (chapter 13)

Chapter 13: Peroneal Muscle Group

(Peroneus Longus, Peroneus Brevis, Peroneus Tertius)

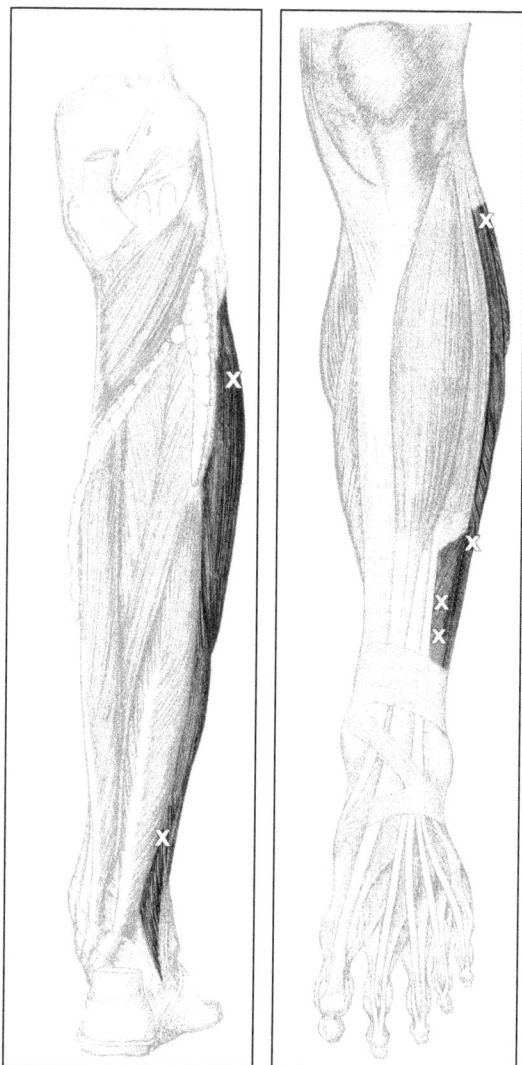

Back view of leg

Front view of leg

Common Symptoms

- the *peroneus longus* and *brevis* refer pain and tenderness over and around the outside ankle bone, over a small area on the outside of your foot, and possibly over a small area over the outside of your lower leg
- the *peroneus tertius* refers pain and tenderness more toward the front of your ankle and possibly behind the outside ankle bone and down toward over your heel
- you may have weak ankles, which are easily broken or sprained over the outside of your ankle
- you may have difficulty in-line or ice skating, unless your boots are very stiff
- if the deep peroneal nerve is entrapped, you may trip frequently due to an inability to lift your foot
- because of the tenderness and pain in and around the ankle joint, trigger point referral can get mis-diagnosed as arthritis
- entrapment of the common peroneal nerve, superficial peroneal nerve, or deep peroneal nerve can cause pain and odd sensations (such as numbness) of the front of your ankle and foot, accompanied by weakness of the ankle

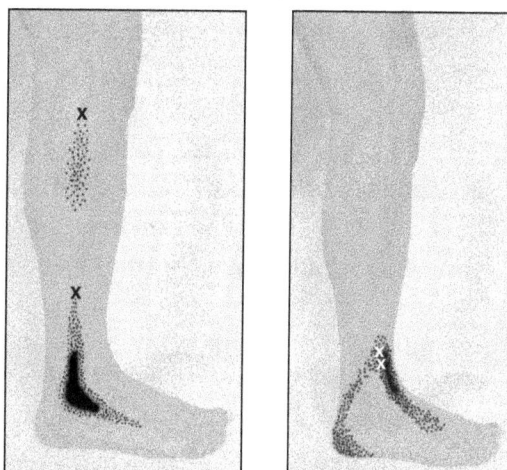

Causes and Perpetuation of Trigger Points

- sprains or fractures in your lower leg, ankle, or foot
- immobilization with a cast
- a longer second toe
- one leg anatomically shorter than the other
- referred pain from trigger points in the *gluteus minimus* (anterior portion, chapter 4)
- associated trigger points in the *tibialis anterior* (chapter 14) and *tibialis posterior* (chapter 12)
- sleeping with your toes pointed
- wearing high heels or shoes with a spike heel of any height
- crossing one leg over the other can compress the common peroneal nerve
- wearing socks or knee-high hose with an elastic band that is too tight

This is a list of perpetuating factors specific only to trigger points in <u>these</u> muscles. For a full list of perpetuating factors that can cause and perpetuate trigger points anywhere in the body and which also apply to these muscles, please see "Appendix A" (found at the end of this book), since some may need to be addressed for lasting pain relief.

Helpful Hints

- If you have pain remaining after a broken leg, ankle, or foot, try searching for trigger points in these muscles, since immobilization with a cast will cause **trigger points.**
- If your socks or hose leave a mark or indentation on your skin from the elastic band, the elastic is too tight and is cutting off needed circulation. Buy socks and hose with a wider, looser band.
- If your foot supinates due to a longer second toe (you will see excessive wear on the outside edge of the heel of your shoe), you will need to get corrective orthotics.
- Don't wear spiked or high heels. Avoid shoes with pointed toes and inadequate room across the top of your toes. Your feet get wider as you get older, and shoes that may once have fit properly may now be too narrow. Any shoes that don't fit or are worn unevenly on the bottoms should be discarded. Buy shoes that have wide soles such as athletic shoes, and get an orthotic insert with a deep heel cup and good arch support (most shoes made these days have minimal or no arch support).
- Walk or run on smooth, level surfaces until trigger points are relieved. Avoid slanted sidewalks, roads or tracks.
- Crossing one leg over the other to compensate for a small hemipelvis (either the right or left half of the pelvis) can compress the common peroneal nerve. If one leg is anatomically shorter than the other, you may have pain on only one side, even if you have a longer second toe on both sides. This is because your weight is shifted to the shorter side, causing a chronic overload of the muscles on that side. The leg may be "shorter" due to foot pronation and a low arch on the affected side rather than an unequal leg bone length. You will need to see a specialist for corrective orthotics or compensating lifts and pads for any of these conditions.
- "Lateral compartment syndrome" is where increased pressure within the muscle compartment adversely affects blood and lymph circulation of the muscles inside (the

peroneus longus and *peroneus brevis*). See the discussion on" Compartment Syndrome" in chapter 1; it is important to see a doctor *immediately* if you have this condition. Lateral compartment syndrome is likely to develop in runners who pronate and have abnormally mobile subtalar joints or if the *peroneus longus* muscle ruptures. Once successfully treated, you should subsequently check for trigger points, since they were likely formed as a result of lateral compartment syndrome.

Self-Help Techniques

Be sure to also search for trigger points in the *gluteus minimus* (chapter 4), *tibialis anterior* (chapter 14) and *tibialis posterior* (chapter 12) muscles for trigger points since they are often the cause of *peroneal* muscle trigger points.

Applying Pressure

Do not apply pressure to your legs if you have varicose veins in the area to be treated -- it could release a clot that could go to your heart or brain! *An acupuncturist or massage therapist should treat your legs, because they can avoid the veins.* You may still do the stretches below.

Gluteus Minimus Pressure: Check the *gluteus minimus* first (anterior portion, chapter 4), since the referred pain can cause satellite trigger points in the *peroneal* muscles.

Peroneal Pressure: Lay on your side on your bed, with a tennis ball between the bed and the side of your lower leg, using gravity for pressure. You can move your leg over the ball to reposition it, but be sure to hold trigger points for eight seconds to one minute, following the general guidelines for self-help found in chapter 2.

Then sit up with your leg out to the side on the bed, and use the thumb or fingers of the same side to check for trigger points in the *peroneus tertius*, one to two inches above the outside ankle bone and closer toward the front of the leg.

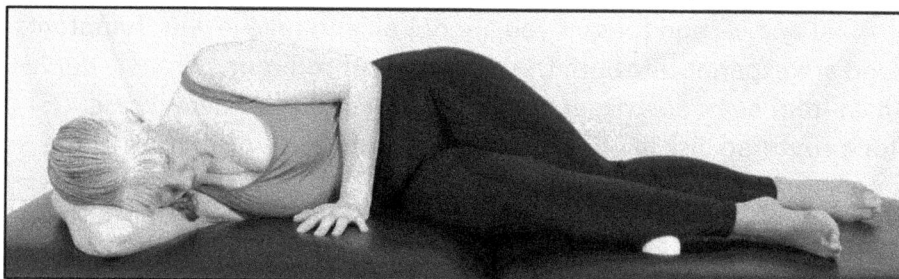

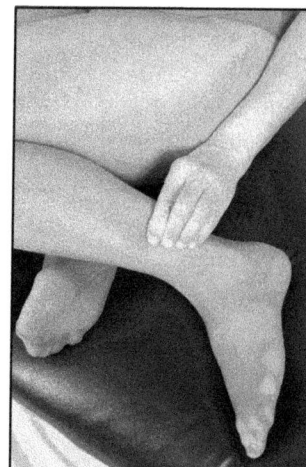

Stretches

Peroneal Stretch: If you are stretching the left side, bring the left foot onto your right thigh. Rotate your foot so the bottom is toward the ceiling. You should feel the stretch on the outside of your lower leg. This is most effective in a hot bath.

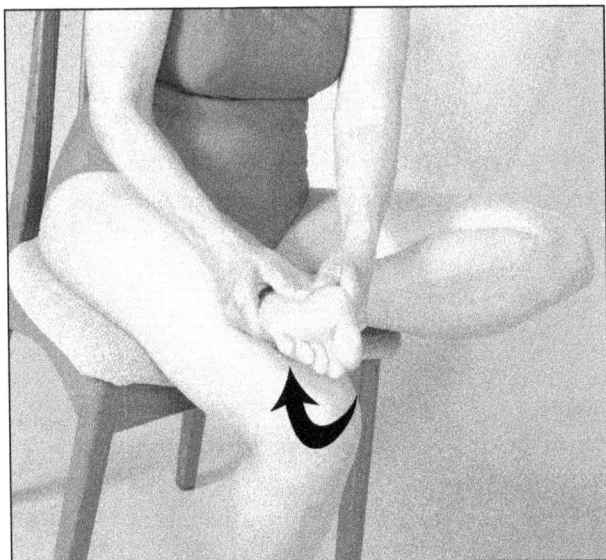

Also See:
* Gluteus minimus (anterior portion, chapter 4)
* Tibialis anterior (chapter 14)
* Tibialis posterior (chapter 12)
* Extensor digitorum longus (chapter 16)

Differential Diagnosis: Trigger points in the *peroneus longus* can entrap the common peroneal nerve on the side of the leg just below the crease of the knee, and weaken both the anterior and lateral compartment muscles. Loss of sensation from the entrapment is greatest in the triangular web between the first and second toes. If you are not able to relieve your symptoms with self-help techniques and are experiencing both the symptoms of common peroneal nerve entrapment and referred pain from *peroneal* trigger points, you need to see a health care provider to be evaluated for a ruptured disk in your back, some kind of cyst, or rupture of the *peroneus longus* muscle.

and *tertius* (chapter 13), the *flexor hallucis longus* (chapter 15), and the first *interosseous* (chapter 18) muscles.

Applying Pressure

Do not apply pressure to your legs if you have varicose veins in the area to be treated -- it could release a clot that could go to your heart or brain! *An acupuncturist or massage therapist should treat your legs, because they can avoid the veins.* You may still do the stretches below.

Gastrocnemius Pressure: It is essential to do self-help techniques on the calves first, since tightness in those muscles is likely the cause of trigger points in the *tibialis anterior*. If you release the *tibialis anterior* first, it could make the pain in the front of the leg much worse. See chapter 10.

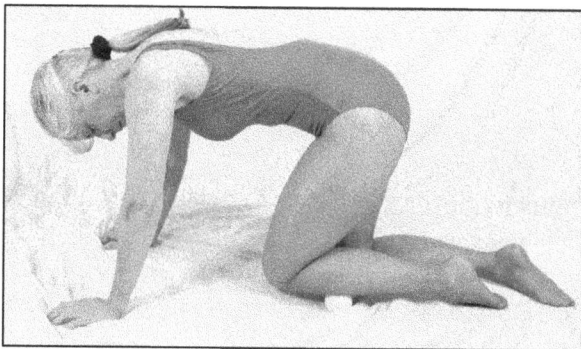

Tibialis Anterior Pressure: Even though most trigger points will be found in the upper 1/3 of the *tibialis anterior*, I like to work the entire length of the muscle. Get down on the floor, and place the tennis ball under the front of your lower leg. The weight of your leg should give you enough pressure. If you need more pressure, shift your weight *toward* the side you are working on. If you need less pressure, shift your weight *away* from the side you are working on. Be sure to keep your head relaxed and let it hang down.

Stretches

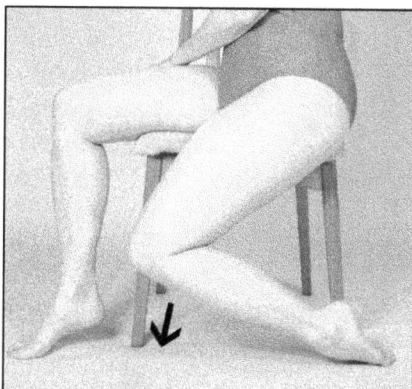

Tibialis Anterior Stretches: Scoot to the edge of a chair, and drop your leg down so your toe is pointing behind you and the top of your foot is on the floor. Press your leg toward the floor until you get a gentle stretch. Adjust the position of your foot until you feel the stretch position that is best for you.

Cross your lower leg over the opposite thigh, and pull the foot and toes back toward you with your hand, so you feel a stretch on the front of your leg. Moving your toes toward the ceiling or the floor will give you a slightly different stretch, so explore which angle is best for you.

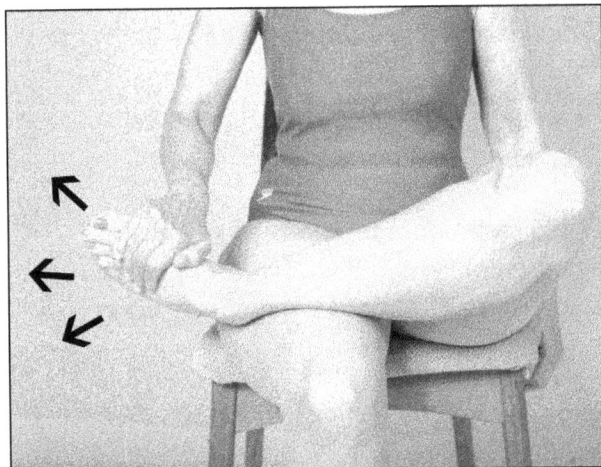

Also See:

* Extensor hallucis longus, extensor digitorum longus (chapter 16)
* Extensor digitorum brevis, extensor hallucis brevis (chapter 17)
* Peroneus tertius, peroneus longus (chapter 13)
* Flexor hallucis longus (chapter 15)
* First interosseous (chapter 18)

Differential Diagnosis: If you are unable to relieve your symptoms with trigger point self-help techniques, you may need to see a health care provider to rule out a bunion, anterior compartment syndrome, and herniation of the *tibialis anterior* muscle. See a chiropractor or osteopathic physician to rule out an L$_5$ vertebra or ankle bones out-of-alignment.

Chapter 15: Long Flexor Muscles of the Toes

(Flexor Digitorum Longus, Flexor Hallucis Longus)

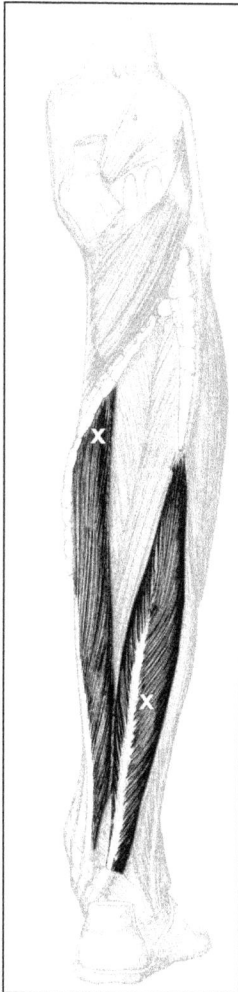

Back view of leg

Hammer toes and clawtoes can form when the *long flexor* muscles of the toes attempt to compensate for a flat foot (pronation). They can also form when the *gastrocnemius* (chapter 10) and *soleus* (chapter 11) are weak (causing the outside and deeper rear calf muscles to try and compensate) combined with a high arch and foot supination, but this is less common. See the discussion in chapter 1.

See Chapter 1 for a discussion of bunions and hallux valgus (the big toe becomes displaced and deformed. Relief of trigger points may stop the progression or even reverse some of the spread of hallux valgus and subsequent bunions, though surgery may be necessary if the condition has progressed far enough.

Common Symptoms

- trigger points in the *flexor digitorum longus* refer pain primarily to the front half of the arch of the foot and into the ball of the foot, and sometimes also into the second through fifth toes, and very occasionally over the inside of the calf and ankle area
- trigger points in the *flexor hallucis longus* refer pain to the bottom of the big toe and the ball of the foot adjacent to the big toe
- pain with walking
- trigger points may occasionally cause painful cramping similar to *gastrocnemius* cramps

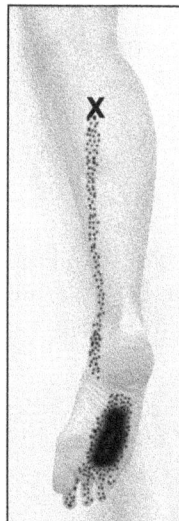

Flexor Digitorum Longus

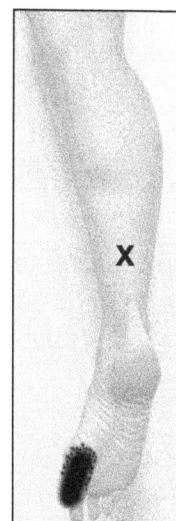

Flexor Hallucis Longus

Causes and Perpetuation of Trigger Points

- walking, running or jogging on uneven ground, sand, or on side-slanted surfaces
- a longer second toe (causing an unstable ankle and foot rocking)
- foot pronation
- continuing to use shoes with worn soles and reduced cushioning
- wearing shoes that aren't very flexible
- weak *gastrocnemius* (chapter 10) and *soleus* (chapter 11) muscles combined with a high arch and foot supination

This is a list of perpetuating factors specific only to trigger points in <u>these</u> muscles. For a full list of perpetuating factors that can cause and perpetuate trigger points anywhere in the body and which also apply to these muscles, please see "Appendix A" (found at the end of this book), since some may need to be addressed for lasting pain relief.

Helpful Hints

- If your ankle is hypo-mobile (doesn't have much movement), see a chiropractor or osteopathic physician to increase mobility. If it is hyper-mobile (moves too much), orthotics with good arch support and a deep heel cup, along with ankle-high shoes for support will help stabilize the foot.
- Wear comfortable shoes with flexible soles and good shock absorption, and make sure they don't cramp your toes, and that the heels aren't too loose. Replace worn shoes, and don't wear high heels.
- Until trigger points are inactivated, walk or run only on smooth surfaces, start with short distances, and increase mileage gradually. Try rowing, swimming, or bicycling instead.
- See the discussion on "Shin Splints" in chapter 1. With these *flexor* muscles, it is now called "medial tibial stress syndrome." At first, pain will be mild and occur later in the exercise, and will be relieved by rest. As this condition progresses, pain will be more intense, occur earlier in the exercise, and may not be relieved once the exercise has stopped. The surface of the bone (periosteum) where the *flexor digitorum longus* attaches on the inside of the lower leg can be loosened and sometimes separated from the deeper part of the bone. A stress fracture can cause similar symptoms.
- The tendon of the *flexor hallucis longus* can rupture spontaneously with overload, without previous injury or disease, and must be repaired surgically.

Self-Help Techniques

Also check the *tibialis posterior* (chapter 12), superficial intrinsic foot muscles (*abductor digiti minimi, flexor digitorum brevis,* chapter 17), and deep intrinsic foot muscles (*adductor hallucis, interossei, flexor hallucis brevis,* chapter 18), since they have similar referral patterns.

Applying Pressure

Do not apply pressure to your legs if you have varicose veins in the area to be treated -- it could release a clot that could go to your heart or brain! *An acupuncturist or massage therapist should treat your legs, because they can avoid the veins.* You may still do the stretches and exercises below.

Gastrocnemius Pressure: The *gastrocnemius* pressure will also treat the *long flexor* muscles of the toes. See chapter 10.

Stretches

Long Flexor Muscles of Toes Stretch: In a seated position, rest your heel on a stool or the floor with your ankle flexed toward your body. With your fingers, pull your toes toward you, and then slowly press your toes away from you, against your fingers. Relax, and repeat.

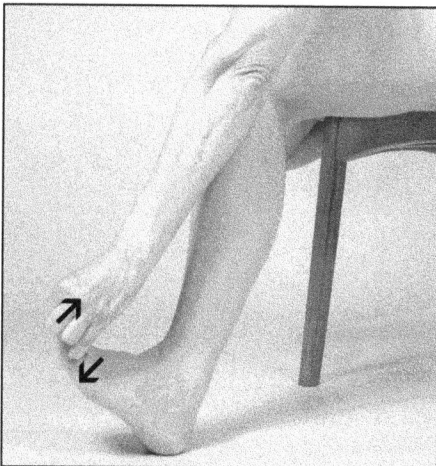

Exercises

Walk in a swimming pool in waist-deep water, taking long strides.

Also See:
* Tibialis posterior (chapter 12)
* Superficial intrinsic foot muscles (chapter 17)
* Adductor hallucis, interossei, flexor hallucis brevis (chapter 18)
* Long extensors of toes (chapter 16)

Differential Diagnosis: Pain on the inside of the ankle from trigger points in the *flexor digitorum longus muscle* can be easily mistaken for pain from tarsal tunnel syndrome. If you are not able to obtain relief with trigger point self-help techniques, you may need to see a health care provider for evaluation for other causes.

Chapter 16: Long Extensor Muscles of the Toes

(Extensor Digitorum Longus, Extensor Hallucis Longus)

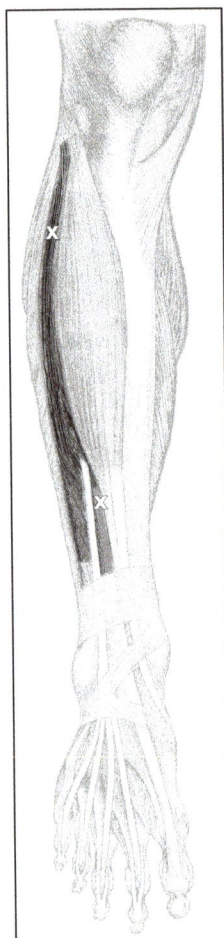

Front view of leg

Chronic tension of the *long extensors* of toes can lead to hammer toe, clawtoe, or mallet toe (see chapter 1 for the discussion). Chronic tension in the *flexor digitorum longus* (chapter 15) and/or weakness in the *lumbricals* (deep muscles on the bottom of the foot, chapter 18) can cause pain in the foot, causing you to lift your foot in a flat manner to avoid forefoot pressure, which overloads the *extensor digitorum longus* muscle. Wearing tight shoes can cause the *lumbricals* to atrophy or fail to develop normally during childhood.

Common Symptoms

- trigger points in the *extensor digitorum longus* refer pain mainly to the top of your foot and over the tops of your three middle toes, and sometimes over the front of your ankle and lower half of the front of your lower leg
- trigger points in the *extensor hallucis longus* refer pain over the top of your foot closest to the big toe, over the top of your big toe, and sometimes over your ankle and a little onto the front of your lower leg
- when walking, the ball of your foot slaps down after heel-strike, or your foot feels "weak"
- trigger points can cause cramps in the front of your lower leg at night, or when your toes are flexed toward your kneecaps for prolonged periods
- "growing pains" in children and adolescents

- the *extensor digitorum longus* can entrap the deep peroneal nerve and cause weakness in the muscles on the front of your lower leg, and an inability to control the upward movement of your forefoot

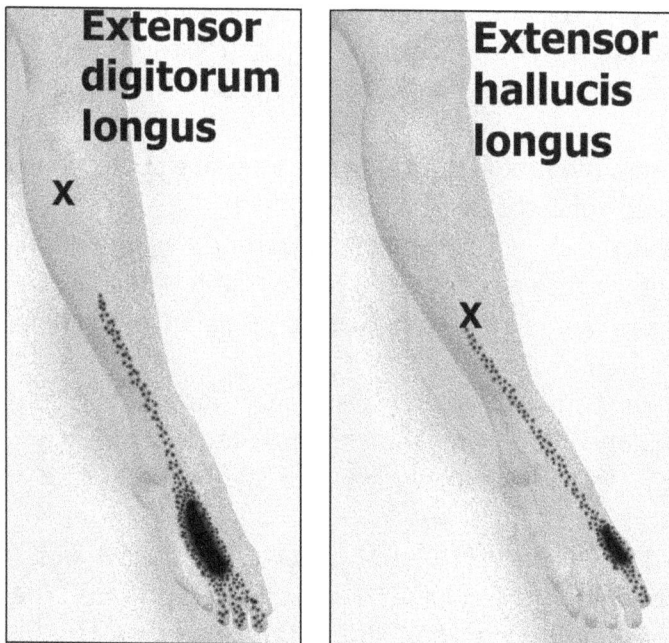

Causes and Perpetuation of Trigger Points

- an L-4 or L-5 nerve root irritation
- tripping or falling
- a direct trauma to the muscle
- a stress fracture in one of the bones of your lower leg
- catching your toe on the ground when kicking a ball
- driving a car with an accelerator pedal that is too vertical or too horizontal
- sitting in a chair with your feet tucked back a bit
- wearing high heels
- tight *gastrocnemius* (chapter 10) and/or *soleus* (chapter 11) muscles which lead to a tight Achilles' tendon, restricting foot movement
- unaccustomed excessive walking, jogging or running, especially on uneven ground
- wearing a cast after a fracture, or immobilization after a sprain
- sleeping with your toes pointed
- anterior compartment syndrome (see the *tibialis anterior*, chapter 14, and "Compartment Syndromes, chapter 1)
- nutritional problems (see perpetuating factors, Appendix A)

This is a list of perpetuating factors specific only to trigger points in <u>these</u> muscles. For a full list of perpetuating factors that can cause and perpetuate trigger points anywhere in the body and which also apply to these muscles, please see "Appendix A" (found at the end of this book), since some may need to be addressed for lasting pain relief.

Helpful Hints

- Wear low heels or flat shoes with a wide base, and get some good orthotics.
- Until trigger points are inactivated, walk or run only on smooth surfaces, start with short distances, and increase mileage gradually. Try rowing, swimming, or bicycling instead.
- When sleeping, keep your feet at a 90-degree neutral angle, with your toes neither pointed nor flexed toward your knees. Try putting a pillow against the bottom of your feet to maintain that position.
- Keep your lower legs warm and covered. Avoid cold drafts, and use a space heater near your legs if necessary. Protect your feet from cold floors.
- If the accelerator pedal in your car is at a steep vertical angle, try putting a wedge on the pedal with the big end at the bottom to reduce the angle of your foot. If it is nearly horizontal, try putting the big end of the wedge at the top. Using cruise control will help. Take breaks every 30-60 minutes.
- If your ankle is hypo-mobile (doesn't have much movement), see a chiropractor or osteopathic physician to increase mobility. If it is hyper-mobile (moves too much), orthotics with good arch support and a deep heel cup, along with ankle-high shoes for support, will help stabilize the foot.
- See the discussions on" Compartment Syndrome" and "Shin Splints" in chapters 1 and 15. It is important to see a doctor *immediately* if you have Compartment Syndrome. The most noticeable symptoms are tightness, dull aching, and diffuse tenderness over the entire belly of the *tibialis anterior* muscle, which is right next to the "shin bone" and runs from below your knee to about three-quarters of the way down the front of your leg.
- Pain from trigger points in the *extensor digitorum longus* muscle may be attributed to pain from the synovial joints in the bones of the foot, so be sure to check for trigger points if you have been given this diagnosis.

Self-Help Techniques

You may also need to check the *peroneal* (chapter 13), *extensor digitorum brevis* (chapter 17), and *interossei* (chapter 18) muscles, since these will also refer pain to the top of the foot, toes and ankle, and are easily confused with referral from trigger points in the *extensor digitorum longus* muscle. Also check the *extensor hallucis brevis* (chapter 17) and *tibialis anterior* (chapter 14) muscles, since trigger point referrals from these muscles are easily confused with those from the *extensor hallucis longus* muscle.

Applying Pressure

Do not apply pressure to your legs if you have varicose veins in the area to be treated -- it could release a clot that could go to your heart or brain! *An acupuncturist or massage therapist should treat your legs, because they can avoid the veins.* You may still do the stretches below.

Long Extensors of Toes Pressure: Get down on the floor on all-fours, and place the tennis ball under the front of your lower leg. The weight of your leg should give you enough pressure. If you need more pressure, shift your weight *toward* the side you are working on. If you need less pressure, shift your weight *away* from the side you are working on. Try to bring your lower leg in toward your body's midline, so you are getting to the front-outside angle of the lower leg.

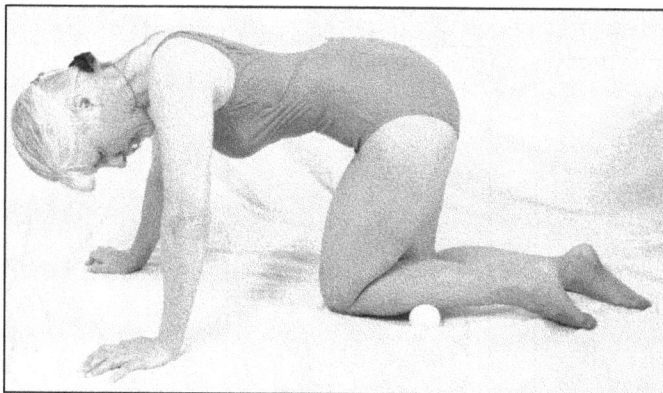

Then lie on your side with the tennis ball under your lower leg, again working toward the front-outside angle of the lower leg (see chapter 13 for the *peroneal* pressure techniques, but try to work farther forward).

Stretches

Tibialis Anterior Stretch: See chapter 14 for these stretches.

Also See:
*   Peroneal (chapter 13)
*   Tibialis anterior (chapter 14)

Differential Diagnosis: Osteoarthritis or possibly other problems may cause inflammation, thinning, and possibly rupture of the extensor hallucis longus tendon, so you may need to see a health care provider for further examination and diagnosis.

Chapter 17: Superficial Intrinsic Foot Muscles

(Extensor Digitorum Brevis, Extensor Hallucis Brevis, Abductor Hallucis,
Flexor Digitorum Brevis, Abductor Digiti Minimi)

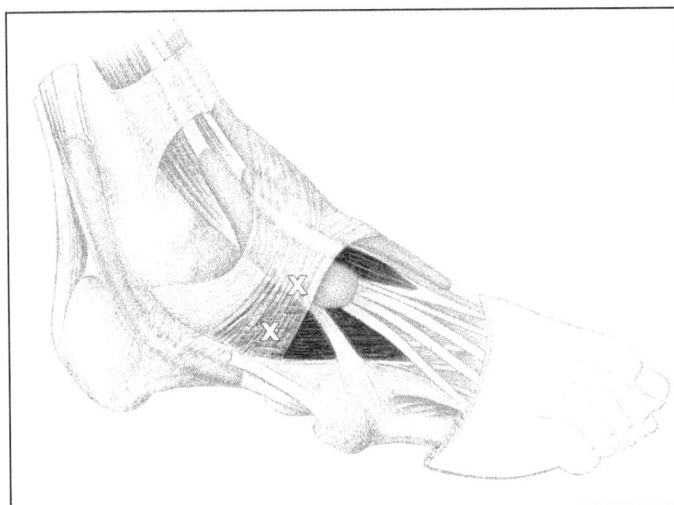

Side of foot

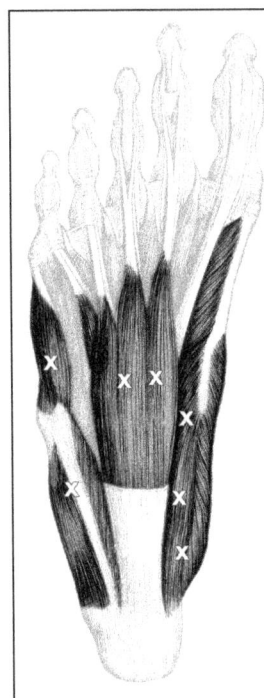

Bottom of foot

Common Symptoms

- pain and tenderness in the foot, but not all the way into the ankle or lower leg
- a tendency to limp and an inability to walk far due to pain
- possibly deep, aching pain even when not using your feet
- orthotics may be uncomfortable if they press against trigger points
- tightness and trigger points can lead to plantar fasciitis, especially when combined with tightness in other muscles
- the *extensor digitorum brevis* and *extensor hallucis brevis* refer pain to the top of the foot, but slightly more toward the outside of the foot
- the *abductor hallucis* refers pain and tenderness mainly to the inside side of the heel, with some spillover pain to the side above the arch and the backside of the heel
- the *abductor digiti minimi* mainly refers pain to the ball of the foot behind the 5th toe, and possibly back a little further onto the sole of the foot
- the *flexor digitorum brevis* refers pain and tenderness to the ball of the foot behind the 2nd, 3rd, and 4th toes, and patients will usually say they have a "sore foot"
- the *abductor hallucis* can entrap the posterior tibial nerve and its two branches, the medial and lateral plantar nerves against the medial tarsal bones, possibly causing tarsal tunnel syndrome

Abductor hallucis

Flexor digitorum brevis

Abductor digiti minimi

Extensors hallucis brevis & digitorum brevis

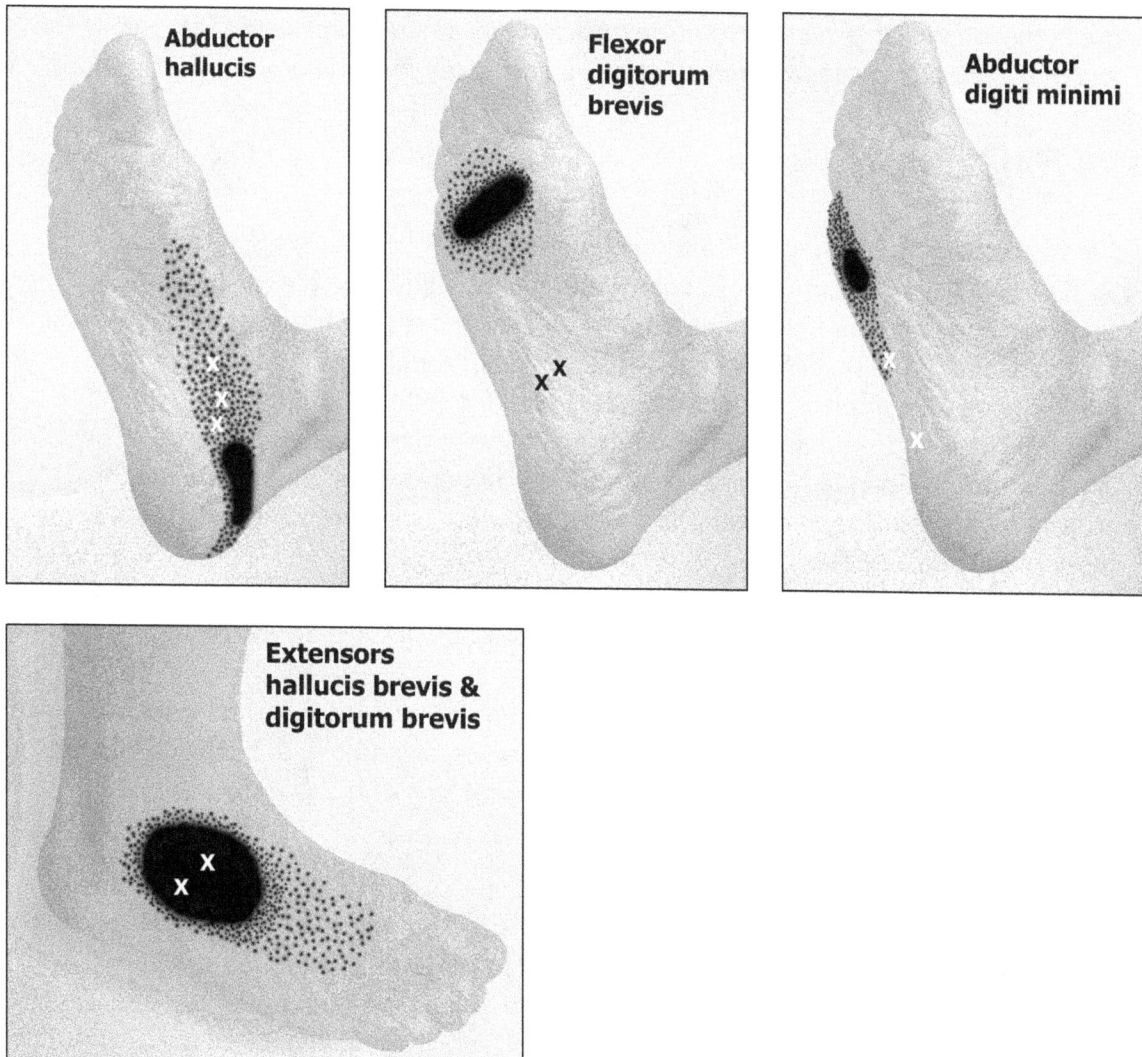

Causes and Perpetuation of Trigger Points

- shoes that are too tight around the toes and ball of your foot
- a fracture of the ankle or other bones of the foot, especially if a cast was used
- injuries by banging or stubbing your toes, or falling
- a longer second toe causing foot rocking can lead to trigger points in the *abductor digiti minimi* and *abductor hallucis muscles*
- foot pronation or supination (standing unevenly on the outside or inside of your feet)
- hypo-mobility or hyper-mobility of the joints of the foot
- inflexible shoes (such as clogs)
- repeatedly using your feet to pull yourself closer to your desk on a rolling chair
- walking or running on uneven ground or a side-slant
- gout (diagnosed with a blood test)

This is a list of perpetuating factors specific only to trigger points in these muscles. For a full list of perpetuating factors that can cause and perpetuate trigger points anywhere in the body and which also apply to these muscles, please see "Appendix A" (found at the end of this book), since some may need to be addressed for lasting pain relief.

Helpful Hints

- See the discussion of plantar fasciitis in chapter 1.
- See chapter 1 for a discussion of bunions and hallux valgus (the big toe becomes displaced and deformed). Relief of trigger points may stop the progression or even reverse some of the spread of hallux valgus and subsequent bunions, though surgery may be necessary if the condition has progressed far enough.
- If your ankle is hypo-mobile (doesn't have much movement), see a chiropractor or osteopathic physician to increase mobility. If it is hyper-mobile (moves too much), orthotics with good arch support and a deep heel cup, along with ankle-high shoes for support will help stabilize the foot.
- Avoid high heels, shoes with narrow toes, and inflexible or slippery soles. Feet get wider and longer with age, so old shoes should be discarded. Pick a shoe with a wide base and cushioning, such as an athletic shoe.
- Until trigger points are inactivated, walk or run only on smooth surfaces, start with short distances, and increase mileage gradually. Try rowing, swimming, or bicycling instead.

Self-Help Techniques

Check the *extensor digitorum longus* (chapter 16) and *peroneus longus* and *brevis* (chapter 13) muscles, since referral patterns are similar to the *extensor hallucis brevis* and *extensor digitorum brevis*. Also check the *adductor hallucis, interossei* (chapter 18), and *flexor digitorum longus* (chapter 15) muscles, since referral patterns are similar to that of the *flexor digitorum brevis*.

Applying Pressure

Plantar Foot Pressure: Sit in a chair and place your foot on top of a golf ball. You may roll it to different spots, holding pressure according to the general guidelines in Chapter 2. Be sure to get into the edge of the arch, and all the way out to the outside edge of the foot. As tenderness decreases, you can use your forearm to lean on your thigh to add pressure. If you need even more pressure, you can stand with your foot resting on the ball, but *do not* shift your weight to that side so that you are actually standing on the ball.

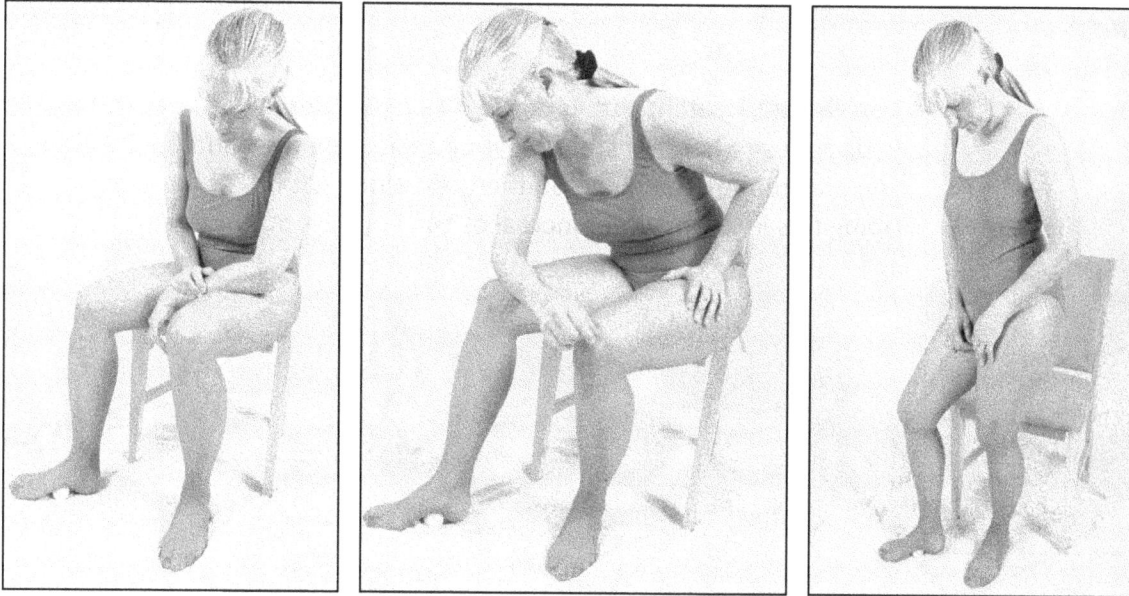

Then sit and bring your foot across the opposite thigh, wrap your hands around your foot, and use one or both thumbs simultaneously to apply massage and pressure to the inside edge of your arch, the area where you cannot reach with the golf ball while your foot is on the floor.

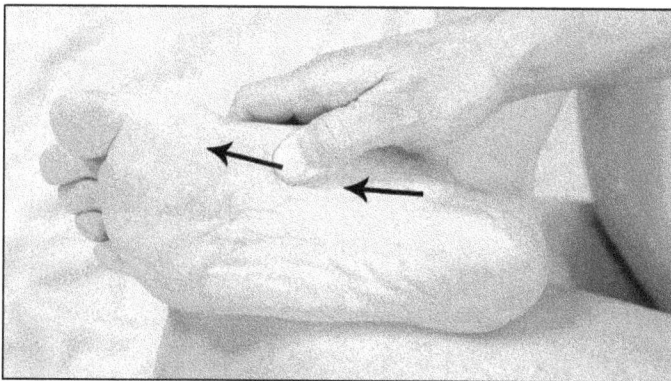

Dorsal Foot Pressure: To treat the *extensors hallucis brevis* and *digitorum brevis*, use your fingers or thumbs on the top of the foot, forward of the outside ankle bone.

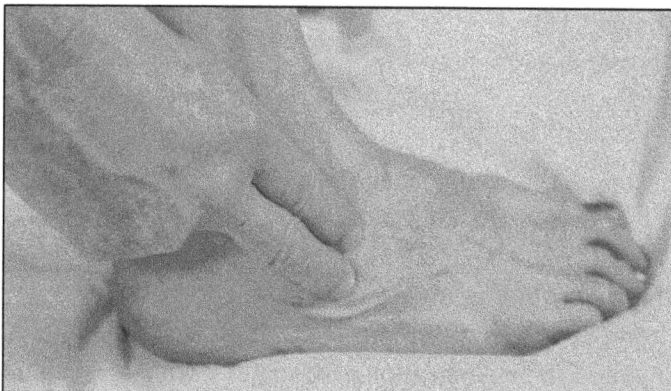

Stretches

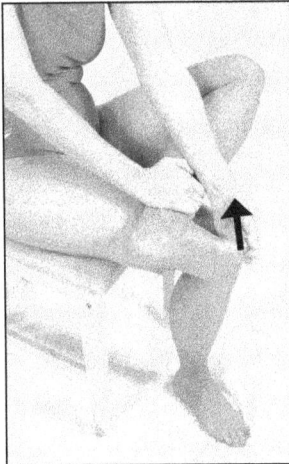

Toe Flexors Stretch: Put your foot over your opposite knee, and use your opposite hand to stabilize your ankle. Use the hand on the side you are treating to pull up on the toes, along with the entire foot. Doing this in warm water increases the benefits of the stretch.

Active Toe Stretch: Sit with your legs stretched out and your heels on the floor. Point your toes while at the same time curling your toes and rotating your feet inward. Then transition to straighten your toes while bringing them up toward your knees and rotating your feet outward. This is a smooth movement. Repeat five times, pausing between each cycle.

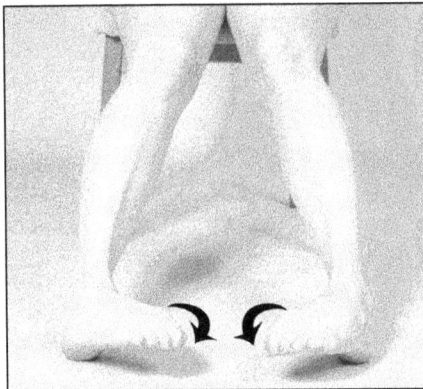

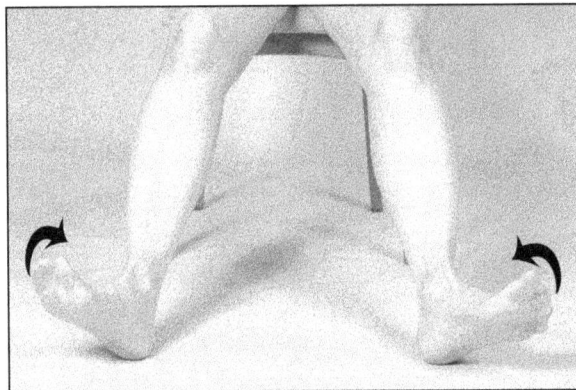

Also See:

* Extensor digitorum longus (chapter 16)
* Peroneus longus and peroneus brevis (chapter 13)
* Adductor hallucis, flexor hallucis brevis, interossei (chapter 18)
* Flexor digitorum longus (chapter 15)
* Gastrocnemius (chapter 10)
* Soleus (chapter 11)
* Quadratus plantae (chapter 18)

Differential Diagnosis: There are many structural problems, such as flat feet, congenital hypertrophy, an avulsion fracture, compartment syndromes, and bones that are out-of-alignment that can cause foot pain. You may need to see a chiropractor, osteopathic physician, or other health care provider to be evaluated for causes of pain other than trigger points.

Chapter 18: Deep Intrinsic Foot Muscles

(Quadratus Plantae and Lumbricals, Flexor Hallucis Brevis,
Adductor Hallucis, Flexor Digiti Minimi Brevis, Interossei)

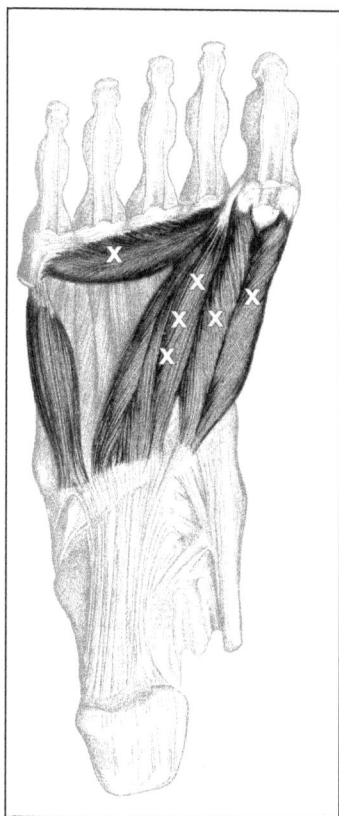

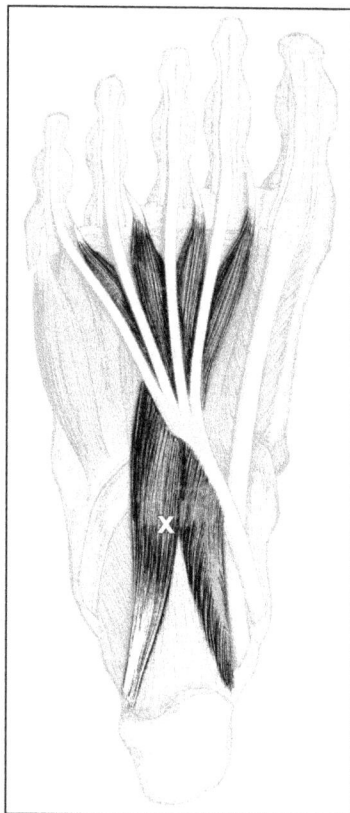

Bottom of foot   *Bottom of foot*   *Center of foot between top and bottom*

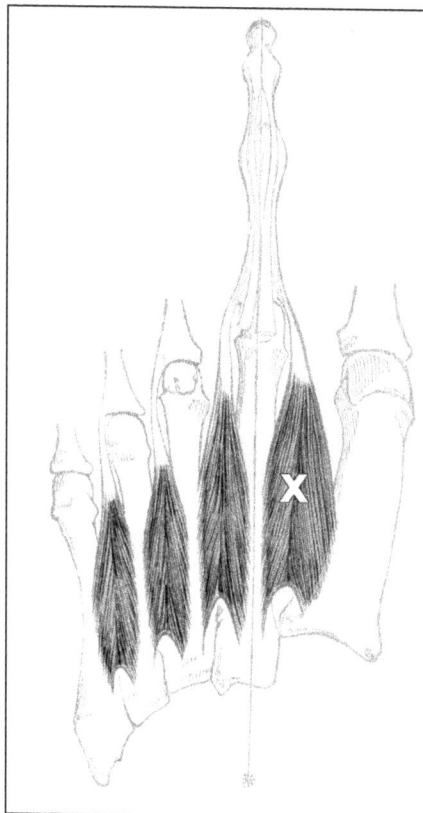

Common Symptoms

- walking is limited due to pain
- numbness of the entire end of the foot accompanied by a feeling of swelling, mostly from trigger points in the *flexor digiti minimi brevis, flexor hallucis brevis,* or *adductor hallucis* muscles
- intolerance to orthotic inserts due to pressure on the trigger points
- the *quadratus plantae* refers pain and tenderness to the bottom of your heel
- the *adductor hallucis* refers pain to the ball of your foot, and is likely to cause a strange "fluffy" feeling of numbness and a sense of swelling of the skin over the ball of the foot
- the *flexor hallucis brevis* refers pain and tenderness on the ball of the foot adjacent to your big toe, on the outside and top of the big toe, with spillover pain that may include most of the second toe
- the *interossei* refer pain down the top of the toe closest to the affected muscle, and on the ball of your foot in a pattern closest to the affected muscle

- the *interosseous* muscle between the 1st and 2nd metatarsals (behind the big and second toes) can cause tingling in the big toe that may also travel into the top of your foot and shin
- trigger points in the *interossei* can cause hammer toes, which may disappear after inactivation of trigger points, particularly in younger patients
- trigger points in the deep intrinsic foot muscles are usually found in combination with trigger points in other muscles that refer pain to the foot

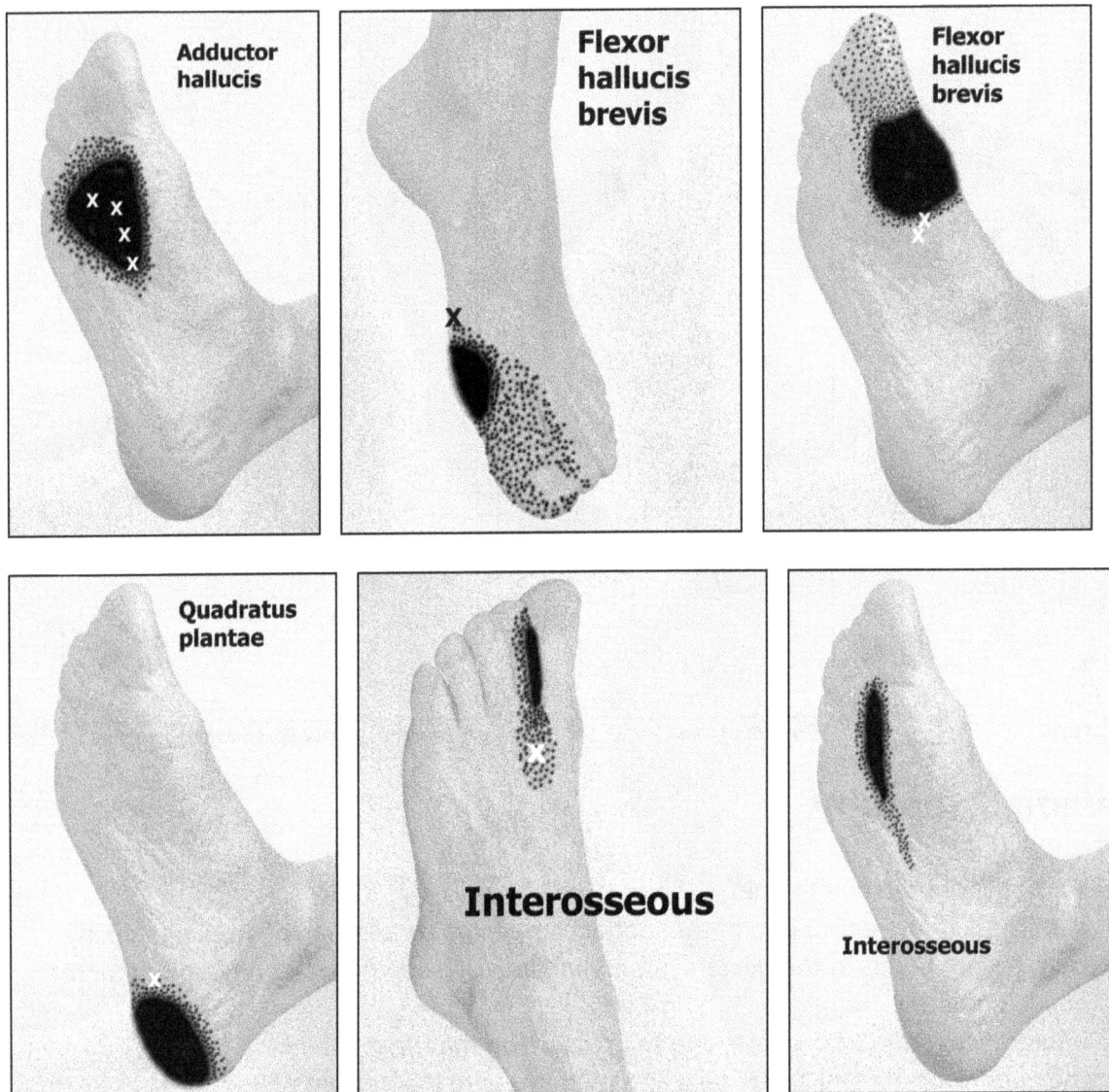

Causes and Perpetuation of Trigger Points

- shoes that are too tight around the toes and ball of your foot
- a fracture of the ankle or other bones of the foot, especially if a cast was used
- injuries by banging or stubbing the toes, or falling
- chilling your feet in cold water or wearing wet socks in cold weather
- a longer second toe causing foot rocking

- foot pronation or supination (standing unevenly on the outside or inside of your feet)
- hypo-mobility or hyper-mobility of the joints of the foot
- inflexible shoes (such as clogs)
- repeatedly using your feet to pull yourself closer to your desk on a rolling chair
- walking or running on uneven ground or a side-slant
- gout (diagnosed with a blood test)

This is a list of perpetuating factors specific only to trigger points in <u>these</u> muscles. For a full list of perpetuating factors that can cause and perpetuate trigger points anywhere in the body and which also apply to these muscles, please see "Appendix A" (found at the end of this book), since some may need to be addressed for lasting pain relief.

Helpful Hints

- The pain and tenderness from *quadratus plantae* trigger points can be confused with plantar fasciitis. See the discussion of plantar fasciitis in chapter 1.
- See chapter 1 for a discussion of bunions and hallux valgus (the big toe becomes displaced and deformed). Relief of trigger points may stop the progression or even reverse some of the spread of hallux valgus and subsequent bunions, though surgery may be necessary if the condition has progressed far enough.
- If your ankle is hypo-mobile (doesn't have much movement), see a chiropractor or osteopathic physician to increase mobility. If it is hyper-mobile (moves too much), orthotics with good arch support and a deep heel cup, along with ankle-high shoes for support will help stabilize the foot.
- Avoid high heels, shoes with narrow toes, and inflexible or slippery soles. Feet get wider and longer with age, so old shoes should be discarded. Pick a shoe with a wide base and cushioning, such as an athletic shoe.
- Until trigger points are inactivated, walk or run only on smooth surfaces, start with short distances, and increase mileage gradually. Try rowing, swimming, or bicycling instead.

Self-Help Techniques

You may need to treat the *extensor digitorum brevis* (chapter 17) and/or *extensor digitorum longus* (chapter 16) first in order to prevent reactive cramping when you release the deep intrinsic foot muscles.

Trigger points in the deep intrinsic foot muscles are usually found in combination with trigger points in other muscles that refer pain to the foot, so be sure to check all the muscles listed in the trigger point location guide for the foot found in chapter 3. Be sure to check the *soleus* (chapter 11), *gastrocnemius* (chapter 10), *flexor digitorum longus* (chapter 15), and *abductor hallucis* (chapter 17), since they can have somewhat similar referral patterns to the *quadratus plantae*. Check the *gastrocnemius* (chapter 10), *flexor digitorum longus* (chapter 15), and the *flexor digitorum brevis* (chapter 17), since referral patterns from those trigger points can be confused with those of the *adductor hallucis*. Check the *tibialis anterior* (chapter 14), *extensor hallucis longus* (chapter 16), and *flexor hallucis longus* (chapter 15), since those trigger points could be confused with referral patterns for the *flexor hallucis brevis*.

Applying Pressure

Plantar Foot Pressure: See chapter 17.

Interossei Pressure: Buy a pencil eraser that fits on the end of a pencil. Using the tip of the eraser, press in-between the bones of the foot on both the top and the bottom. You may hold pressure, but also move the eraser back and forth in the groove in-between the long bones of the foot.

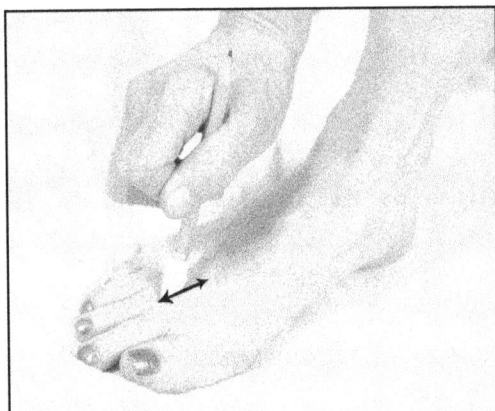

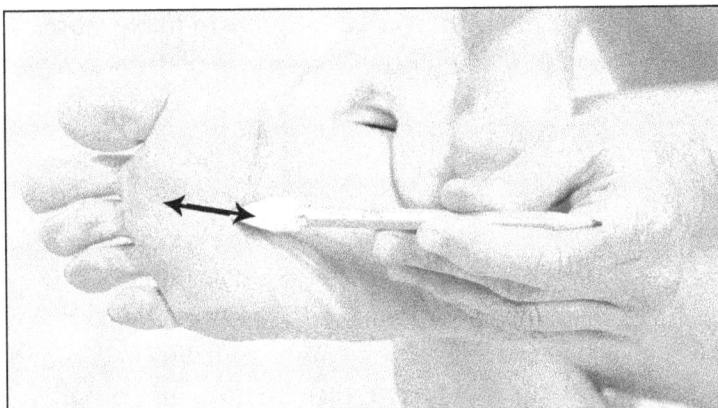

Stretches

The stretches are the same as in chapter 17.

Also See:

*   Soleus (chapter 11)
*   Gastrocnemius (chapter 10)
*   Flexor hallucis longus, flexor digitorum longus (chapter 15)
*   Flexor digitorum brevis, abductor hallucis, (chapter 17)
*   Tibialis anterior (chapter 14)
*   Extensor hallucis longus (chapter 16)

Differential Diagnosis: If you are unable to relieve your symptoms with trigger point self-help techniques, you may need to see a health care provider to rule out stress fractures of the foot, structural deviations, or an injury to a sesamoid bone (the little bones on the ball of the foot at the base of the big toe) in the flexor hallucis brevis tendon.

Anyone with sore intrinsic foot muscles, particularly associated with inflammation of the big toe joints, should be tested for gout and subsequently managed, in order to obtain lasting relief with trigger point therapy.

APPENDIX A

What Causes and Keeps Trigger Points Going: Perpetuating Factors

"If we treat myofascial pain syndromes without . . . correcting the multiple perpetuating factors, the patient is doomed to endless cycles of treatment and relapse. [Perpetuating factors are] the most neglected part of the management of myofascial pain syndromes . . . The answer to the question, 'How long will the beneficial results of specific myofascial therapy last?', depends largely on what perpetuating factors remain unresolved . . . One may view perpetuating factors also as predisposing factors, since their presence tends to make the muscles more susceptible to the activation of [trigger points] . . . Usually, one stress activates the [trigger point], then other factors perpetuate it. In some patients, these perpetuating factors are so important that their elimination results in complete relief of the pain without any local treatment." ~~ *Doctors Janet Travell and David G. Simons*

There is much more to "Neuromuscular Therapy" or "Trigger Point Therapy" than learning referral patterns and how to search for trigger points; it is very important for a health care provider to identify and figure out *with* the patient what is causing and perpetuating their symptoms. This requires getting a complete medical history and evaluating for any potential perpetuating factors.

Trigger points are a *symptom*, not a *cause*. Needling or applying pressure to the trigger points treats the acute part of the problem, but does not resolve the underlying factors. If you get temporary relief from trigger point therapy but symptoms quickly recur, then trigger points are definitely a factor, but perpetuating factors need to be addressed in order to gain lasting relief.

This appendix will outline some general causes of trigger point activation and how to address the factors, and each muscle chapter will specifically address issues particularly pertinent to that muscle. I recommend you read all of the perpetuating factors, since you likely have more than one factor that you may not have recognized up to this point.

Acute or Chronic Viral, Bacterial, and Parasitic Infections

Acute infections, such as **colds, flu, strep throat, and bronchitis** will aggravate trigger points, particularly in a person with fibromyalgia or chronic fatigue. It is important to head off illness at the first sign in order to avoid perpetuating trigger points. When you start to get sick, take the Chinese herbs Gan Mao Ling or Yin Chiao, Echinacea, and/or homeopathics such as Osillococcinum or other appropriate homeopathics for colds, flu, or sinusitis. Once you are past the initial stage of illness, if symptoms progress, the Chinese herbs you take will be determined by your particular set of symptoms, so at this point you may need professional help to determine the proper herbs. You should have the above-mentioned herbs and homeopathics available at home so you can treat your symptoms as soon as you notice the first signs. This is particularly important if you have fibromyalgia, sinusitis, asthma, or other recurrent infections, since your trigger points will be activated by illness, and getting sick can set you back by weeks in your treatment and healing.

Outbreaks of **chronic infections**, such as **herpes simplex** (cold sores, genital herpes, herpes zoster) will also aggravate trigger points, and may need to be managed if recurrence is frequent. There are many pharmaceutical drugs and natural supplements/herbs for treating recurrent herpes infections, and some will work better than others for you. Also, if you are getting recurrent outbreaks you will want figure out what is stressing your immune system, such as allergies or emotional stress. Sometimes a herpes outbreak is the first sign you are fighting an acute illness, so that is the time to take the above-mentioned supplements.

Other chronic infections such as **sinus infections, an abscessed or impacted tooth, or urinary tract infections** will perpetuate trigger points. If you suspect a **tooth**, you will need to see your dentist for evaluation. **Urinary tract infections** (UTI's) need to be dealt with promptly. You may use over-the-counter western drugs, Chinese herbs, and cranberry (don't use sweetened juice), but if you don't respond to treatment immediately you will need to see your health care provider, since UTI's can turn into life-threatening kidney infections. Any mechanical reasons for **sinus infections** need to be dealt with for lasting relief. Naturopathic doctors can use a small inflatable balloon to open up the passages. You may need surgical intervention if the blockage is severe enough. Many people report success using a Neti Pot (get it at your health food store) to flush the sinuses with a warm saline solution. With both sinus infections and UTI's, antibiotics often won't kill all of the pathogens, and you may get a lingering, recurrent infection. However, antibiotics also work quickly, so I often recommend to patients that they combine antibiotics, acupuncture, herbs, and homeopathics to knock the infection out as quickly and completely as possible so it doesn't become a chronic problem.

The fish tapeworm, giardia, and occasionally amoeba are the most likely **parasites** to perpetuate trigger points. The fish tapeworm and giardia scar the lining of the intestine and impair your ability to absorb nutrients, and they also consume vitamin B-12. **Amoeba** can produce toxins that are passed from the intestine into the body. **Fish tapeworms** can be transmitted from raw fish. **Giardia** is most often associated with drinking untreated water from streams, but it can also be passed by an infected person not washing their hands after a bowel movement, particularly if they are preparing food or have some other hand-to-mouth contact.

Any time you have **chronic diarrhea** it is worth testing for parasites. A cheaper alternative is just to treat with herbs like grapefruit seed extract or Pulsatilla (a Chinese herb) and see if your symptoms improve. Since these will also kill off the good intestinal flora, you will want to follow treatment with a good multi-acidophilus supplement, as you would after any antibiotic. If you have blood in your stools, you should always see your health care provider immediately to rule out serious conditions. Acupuncture and Naturopathy can help resolve chronic diarrhea from most causes.

There is substantial controversy about whether **systemic candida infections** exist, though it is now listed in the Merck Manual (a medical text of illness and disease). There is abundant information on the Web regarding this subject, so I won't go into detail. Candida is a normal intestinal flora, but can multiply beyond a normal amount and cause a variety of symptoms including muscular pain. Many people report feeling much better on an anti-candida diet, and in any case it is a pretty healthy way to eat. There are many herbal products on the market for eliminating candida, including grapefruit seed extract, oil of oregano, Echinacea, Pulsatilla, and many formulas. Again, you will want to follow any of these with a good multi-acidophilus supplement to replace the beneficial intestinal flora.

Allergies and other Environmental Stressors

Both inhaled and ingested allergens perpetuate trigger points and make them harder to treat due to the subsequent histamine release. Skin tests are useful for testing for **inhaled allergens**, and there are a few methods for testing for **food allergens**.

One of the best ways to test for **food allergens** is an elimination diet, where you eliminate all foods, add them back in one at a time, and then rotate foods. You can find instructions for this in *"Prescription for Nutritional Healing"* by Balch and Balch under "Allergies." The challenge with a rotation diet is that most people are not willing to do it, as it takes a very strict control of your diet and a careful food diary for a month. As an alternative, Balch and Balch offer a quick-test. After sitting and relaxing for a few minutes, take your pulse rate for one minute, then eat the food you are testing. Keep still for 15-20 minutes and take your pulse again. If your pulse rate has increased more than ten beats per minute, eliminate this food from your diet for one month, then re-test. Naturopathic doctors offer a blood test for food sensitivities. Food allergens and sensitivities must be eliminated, but this can become challenging when you eat at other people's homes, when dining out, or while traveling. Try to keep something you *can* have with you, so you have an alternative.

There may be some ingested substances to which you are not allergic, but can aggravate your condition anyway and should be avoided. Chinese diagnosis differentiates pain by the quality of the pain (dull, achy, sharp, shooting, stabbing, burning, moving) and what makes it better or worse (i.e., rest/activity, heat/cold/damp, etc.), and some foods will aggravate certain conditions. You can see an Oriental Medicine practitioner for an evaluation of your pain and to get dietary advice, but you can try eliminating the following foods to see if it helps: coffee and black tea (yes, even decaf!), alcohol, bananas, peanuts, dairy, greasy foods, pop, sugar, wheat, and spicy foods.

Environmental allergies must be controlled as much as possible, and if you see a specialist for a skin test to identify allergens, they will make specific suggestions based on the allergen. A good HEPA air filter will help substantially, and you will need one for each room. Make sure each unit is large enough to cover the needed square footage. Not all air filters are equal, so be sure to research your options. An ozonator will kill molds, but I do not suggest leaving one running while you or pets are in the room, even though some are made for that purpose. Get an ozonator that puts out enough ozone that you can "bomb" the room while you and your pets are gone. Bomb one room at a time and close the door so that you will get a high concentration. After a few hours, hold your breath and open the windows and let the room air out for a couple of minutes before you occupy the room again. You will smell ozone (like lightening) lingering, but the air is fine to breathe after just a few minutes, so don't be concerned.

Seasonal Affective Disorder (SAD) affects millions of people to one degree or another, particularly people living closer to the North or South poles where the daylight hours are shorter in winter. SAD causes symptoms such as depression, loss of energy, decreased activity, fatigue, sleeping up to four extra hours per night, irritability and crying spells, difficulty concentrating, carbohydrate cravings, and increased appetite and weight gain. Though SAD probably does not directly cause pain, many of these symptoms *can* contribute to pain eventually. For example, if increased activity helps reduce your pain but SAD keeps you from exercising, then the SAD needs to be treated in order to help reduce your pain. Most SAD patients improve when they get additional light in their retinas. Unless you sit right next to a window in your office, you are probably not getting enough light. You may be traveling to and from work in the dark much of the year. One solution is to make sure you get outside during daylight hours, possibly for a walk at your lunch hour. Another solution is to buy a therapeutic light box. Full-spectrum lights alone are not strong enough to be of therapeutic value, so you need to get a box with reflective materials capable of producing 10,000 LUX. You need to be within 24" of the box in most cases (the light box should come with instructions that tell you how close you need to be to get 10,000 LUX), and you need to have your eyes open and looking toward the box so you get the light in your retinas.

   Toxic metals exposure has been implicated in pain syndromes. A hair analysis obtained through a naturopathic doctor can evaluate toxic levels of chemicals and mineral levels. If you find you have high levels of toxic metals, the doctor can help you with a detox program.

Emotional Factors

   While it is important to recognize the role of stress and emotional factors in creating and perpetuating illness, unfortunately all too often patients are dismissed (or medicated) by their health care providers as "just being under stress." They depart the health care provider's office with their physical symptoms not being assessed or addressed, particularly when it comes to the symptoms of pain and depression. This seems to happen more frequently to women, but I've also had male patients who had the same experience.

   Antidepressants are often prescribed, which may possibly help with the acute symptoms, but the side-effects can add to the underlying condition causing the symptoms, and a vicious cycle ensues. If you are in pain long enough, of *course* you will begin to get fatigued and depressed. If you are depressed long enough, you will probably develop pain. Anything that has gone on long enough *will* have both components.

   One of the things I like most about Oriental Medicine and homeopathy is that both modalities assume you cannot separate the physical body from the emotions, and symptoms of both are used to develop a diagnosis, and are treated simultaneously. With acupuncture there are no side-effects, and response is usually rapid. With both homeopathy and herbs (Chinese or American) the wrong prescription or dosage can have side-effects, just as with Western prescription drugs, so it is important to consult with a trained professional.

   If you are **angry, anxious or stressed**, chances are you are holding at least some of your body parts very tense, and developing trigger points. You may be hiking your shoulders up around your neck, tightening your forearms or abdomen, or tensing your gluteal muscles (women tense their gluteal muscles more often than men). In addition to dealing with the underlying cause of emotional factors, you will have to notice when you are tensing body parts, and keep consciously relaxing them over and over again. You are re-training yourself to not tense your muscles. Bio-feedback can help with this.

If you are experiencing an unusual desire to be alone, a disinterest in your favorite activities, a decrease in job performance, and are neglecting your appearance and hygiene, you may be suffering from **depression**. Other symptoms of depression are insomnia, loss of appetite, weight loss, impotence or a lowered libido, blurred vision, a sad mood, thoughts of suicide or death, an inability to concentrate, a poor memory, indecision, mumbled speech, and negative reactions to suggestions. No one symptom will confirm a diagnosis of depression, because there are other reasons for some of these symptoms. It is the combination of symptoms that confirms a depression diagnosis. Depression lowers your pain threshold, increases pain, and adversely affects your response to trigger point therapy. (See the section on Organ Dysfunction and Disease, **thyroid**, below, since thyroid problems can be an undiagnosed cause of depression.)

If you are angry, depressed, anxious, or stressed, you will need to address this in some manner in order to speed recovery from pain. Often people suffering from severe emotional factors, chronic fatigue and/or extreme pain lack the energy to participate in their own healing. You may have difficulty feeding yourself properly or even getting out of bed, and cannot manage even mild forms of exercise such as walking -- the very things that would help you start to feel better. You may have difficulty making it to your appointments. If this describes you, you will need to do *whatever you can* to get to the point where you can start taking better care of yourself. This may mean getting antidepressants, acupuncture, homeopathy, counseling, pain relievers, and/or doing the self-help techniques in this book. Walking and deep breathing are great tension and depression-relievers. Even walking ten minutes per day (especially outside) can be extremely beneficial. Just doing one of these things will help get you started in the right direction and improve your energy and outlook.

"Secondary Gains"

Sometimes we subconsciously get something out of being sick or in pain. For example, if you have a hard time saying "no," it is easier to excuse yourself by not feeling well, rather than having to bear the brunt of the reactions you get from people who aren't used to you refusing their requests or demands. Some people have a need to stay in pain in order to get attention. Perhaps in childhood that was the only way they could get their parent's attention and they are still using that strategy as an adult. Sometimes it's easier to focus on physical symptoms than deal with underlying anxiety and emotional problems. Some people have financial reasons for not getting well, such as disability payments or lawsuit settlements, or it may get them out of some things they don't want to do.

If you find yourself complaining about your physical symptoms but not doing anything to relieve them, you might want to ask yourself what you may be getting out of staying sick. This is not always the case, as in severe depression, but it is worth at least exploring. Chances are, if you have purchased this book, you do not have subconscious needs to stay sick or in pain, since you have already taken a step to help yourself.

Good Sport Syndrome

Many people believe in pushing through the pain -- that it will make them stronger and is beneficial. Wrong! This just aggravates existing problems and makes them harder to treat. Exercise should be comfortable, such as alternating running with walking or resting in between weight repetitions, and using weights that aren't too heavy. If you tend to overdo things, you will need to back off on your activities and add them back in slowly with the guidance of your practitioner. Returning to activities too soon or excessively will quickly wipe out your therapeutic progress.

Injuries

A healthy muscle is pliable to the touch when it is not being used, but will feel firm if called upon for action. If a muscle feels firm at rest, it is tight in an unhealthy way (even if you work-out). I like to use an analogy of a rubber band or stick. Imagine that a sudden, unexpected force is applied to the "stick," or tight muscle (such as a fall). Like a stick, the muscle will be damaged. If a sudden force is applied to a pliable muscle, or "rubberband," it will stretch with the force instead, and will be much less likely to be injured. Since latent trigger points restrict range-of-motion to some degree, and almost everyone has some latent trigger points, a muscle may be tight and restricted without you being aware of it, and can be easily injured if a sudden force is applied.

Injuries are one of the most common initiators of trigger points. **People who exercise regularly are less likely to develop trigger points** than those who exercise occasionally and overdo it. If you have an injury, begin treatment as soon as possible. Apply cold during the first 48 hours, and use some form of arnica homeopathic orally and/or topically as soon as possible. There are Chinese herb formulas for trauma that you can get from an acupuncturist or possibly a health food store. Have these available in your medicine cabinet since it may be hard for you to go to the store after you are injured, and because these work best when started immediately after the injury. See an acupuncturist or massage therapist who is experienced in working with recent injuries. You may also need to see a chiropractor, osteopathic physician, or physical therapist.

Surgeries will likely leave some amount of scar tissue, which can perpetuate trigger points in adjacent muscle fibers. **Scar tissue** can be broken up to an extent with cross-friction massage. Because this is usually fairly painful, I only work on scars for a few minutes each appointment, and I warn the patient that it will be painful but that I won't do it for more than a few minutes. Most patients will not work on their own scars vigorously enough due to the pain level. Acupuncture can treat scar tissue and help eliminate the pain from trigger points around the area. I recommend using both cross-friction massage and acupuncture as part of the treatment protocol, rather than just one or the other.

Mechanical Stresses

Chronic mechanical stresses are one of the most common causes of trigger point activation and perpetuation, and are nearly always correctable. A **skeletal asymmetry**, including an anatomically shorter leg and a small hemipelvis (either the right or left half of the pelvis) can be corrected with shoe lifts and butt lifts. [NOTE: In this book, reference to a "shorter leg" refers to a *true* anatomical leg length inequality where the bones are shorter on one side, rather than the "shorter leg" caused by a spinal mis-alignment, which is a term chiropractors use.] A **skeletal disproportion**, such as a long second toe can be corrected with shoe orthotics, and short upper arms can be corrected with ergonomically correct furniture. Vertebral subluxation and other bones-out-alignment can be adjusted by a chiropractor or osteopathic physician, especially if the muscles are also first relaxed by an acupuncturist or massage therapist. Your physical therapist may be trained in manipulations.

Wearing appropriate shoes can help relieve symptoms in your entire body (see "Abuse of Muscles," below). **Orthotics** can help even more. My favorite non-corrective orthotics are the Superfeet brand. They have a deep heel cup which helps prevent pronation (more weight on the inside of your foot) and supination (more weight on the outside of the foot), and they have excellent arch support. Superfeet has a variety of models, including cheaper non-custom "Trim-to-Fit" footbeds, and moderately-priced custom molded footbeds to provide support in a variety of footwear. See Superfeet.com to learn more about their products. If you find you need corrective orthotics, you will need to see a podiatrist. If you decide to get custom orthotics, be sure to work on your trigger points first, because as the muscles relax you will stand differently and the orthotics need to be formed for the corrected stance.

Misfitting furniture is a major cause of muscular pain, particularly in the work place. There are companies that specialize in coming into your work place and correcting your office arrangement, and fitting you for furniture that fits your body. Your employer may balk at the cost, but if they don't change your misfitting furniture, they will end up paying for it in lost work time and worker's compensation claims.

I see a lot of what I call "mouse injuries" -- arm and shoulder pain due to using a computer mouse for extended periods of time without proper arm support. The keyboard should be kept as close to lap level as possible. When not using your computer, your elbows and forearms should rest evenly on either your work surface or armrests of the proper height. Your computer screen should be directly in front of you with the middle of the screen slightly below eye level, and the copy attached to the side of the screen, so that you may look directly forward as much as possible. Your knees should fit under your desk, and the chair needs to be close enough that you can lean against your backrest. A good chair will have a backrest with a slope of 25 to 30-degrees back from the vertical which supports both the lumbar area and the mid-back. The seat should be low enough that your feet rest flat on the floor without compression of the thigh by the front edge of the seat, high enough that not all the pressure is put on the buttocks, and slightly hollowed out to accommodate the buttocks. The armrests must be high enough to provide support for the elbows without having to lean to the side, but not so high as to cause the shoulders to hike up. The upholstery needs to be firm and casters should be avoided. I highly recommend headsets for phones to solve neck and back pain.

A lumbar support helps correct round-shouldered posture. Most chiropractic offices carry lumbar supports of varying thickness. I recommend getting one for the car (most car seats actually *curve the wrong way* in the lumbar area) and your favorite seat at home, and investing in a good chair for the office, even if your employer won't. Try to avoid sitting in or on anything without back support, which causes you to sit with your shoulders and upper back slumped forward. When going to sporting events, picnics, or other places you won't have a back support, bring a *Crazy Creek Chair™* (or something similar) to provide at least some support. You can get one through most of the major sporting goods suppliers for about $49, a good investment in your back, and they are very lightweight for carrying. Or consider a lightweight collapsible chair, also available at sporting goods stores.

Sleeping in a sagging bed can cause back and hip problems. (See the section on Sleep Problems below).

But properly fitting furniture won't help as much if you are not also conscientious of avoiding **poor posture**. If you slouch at your desk or on your couch at home, or read in bed, for example, your muscles will suffer. **Abuse of muscles** includes poor body mechanics (i.e., lifting improperly), long periods of immobility (i.e., sitting at a desk without a break), repetitive movements (i.e., computer use), holding your body in an awkward position for long periods (i.e., dentists and mechanics), and excessively quick and jerky movements (i.e., sports). Learn to lift properly and take frequent breaks from anything you must do for long time periods.

If you have a habit of immobilizing your muscles to protect against pain, you will need to start gently increasing your range of motion as you inactivate trigger points. Don't keep stressing the muscles to see if it still hurts or to demonstrate to your treating professionals where you have to move it to in order to get it to hurt -- if you keep repeating this motion, you will just keep the trigger points activated.

Be sure to sit while putting clothing on your lower body. Don't wear high heels or cowboy boots. If you carry a purse, get a strap long enough that you can wear it diagonally across your body, rather than over one shoulder. If you use a day pack, put the straps over both shoulders. Without realizing it, you are hiking up one shoulder at least a little to keep the straps from slipping off no matter *how* light your purse or pack may be. Notice whether you hold your shoulders up or are tightening muscles such as your butt, arms, or abdomen when you are under stress. You will need to re-train yourself to break this habit.

If you are clenching your jaw or grinding your teeth, see a dentist for help. The soft plastic bite splints found over-the-counter in pharmacies are too soft and do not help temporomandibular joint dysfunction. You need to be fitted by your dentist for a hard, slippery acrylic night guard.

Constricting clothing can lead to muscular problems. My rule of thumb is, if the clothing item leaves an elastic mark or indentation in the skin, it is too tight and is cutting off proper circulation. Check your bras, socks, ties, and belts to see if they are too tight.

Be sure to check muscles listed in the muscle chapters that can cause "satellite trigger points," since this is one perpetuating cause. For example, if you find trigger points in the abdominal muscles but trigger points quickly recur, check the paraspinal muscles also, because trigger points there can refer to the abdominal area and cause trigger points to be reactivated.

Nutritional Problems and Diet

Doctors Travell and Simons found that almost half of their patients required treatment for **vitamin inadequacies** to obtain lasting relief from the pain and dysfunction of trigger points, and thought it was one of the most important perpetuating factors to address. They found **the most important were the water-soluble vitamins B-1, B-6, B-12, folic acid, vitamin C, and the minerals calcium, magnesium, iron and potassium**. Other researchers have now added **vitamin D** to that list.

The more deficient in nutrients you are, the more symptoms you will have, and your trigger points and nervous system will be more hyper-irritable. Even if a blood test determines you are at the low end of the normal range, you may still need more of a nutrient, since your body will pull nutrients from the tissues before it will allow a decrease in the blood levels. Several factors may lead to nutrient insufficiency:

- An inadequate intake of a nutrient

- Impaired nutrient absorption
- Inadequate nutrient utilization
- An increased need by the body
- A nutrient leaving the body too quickly
- A nutrient being destroyed within the body too quickly

You may be in a **high risk group** if you are: elderly, pregnant or nursing, an alcoholic or other drug user, poor, depressed, or seriously ill. If you tend to diet by leaving out important food groups, or have an eating disorder, you will also deplete yourself of necessary nutrients.

- Even if you have a fairly healthy diet, because our soils have been depleted in nutrients from too frequent crop-rotations, chemical fertilizers, and long shipping distances, our food does not provide all the nutrition we require. In addition, many of us don't have a very balanced diet, and processed foods do not contain as much nutrition as fresh-prepared. Most people need to take some kind of **multi-supplement** to ensure proper nutrition, especially if you fall into one of the high risk groups mentioned above. Because some vitamins require the presence of other vitamins, a good multi-supplement ensures the needed combination is present. Be sure to check the label to make sure there are adequate minerals in a multi -- you may need to also take a multi-mineral. Improving your nutrient intake to see if it improves your symptoms is an easy and relatively inexpensive therapy to try. Take your vitamins with food, since some need to bind with substances found in food in order to be absorbed.

Building up sufficient levels of vitamin B-12, vitamin D, and iron may take several months; don't get discouraged if you don't see immediate results, though you may start gradually feeling better within a few weeks from taking multivitamin and multimineral supplements.

- You may still need to be tested by a health care provider for inadequacies, since some people are not able to absorb certain nutrients, and need to have them injected or mega-dosed. For example, some people cannot absorb B-12, and need to get intramuscular injections to provide that necessary vitamin.

- **Take your vitamins and herbs when you are *not* sick** -- the germs also like the vitamins and herbs and they will get stronger. See the section above on Acute or Chronic Viral, Bacterial, and Parasitic Infections for suggestions on how to head off illness. Once all symptoms have abated, you may switch back to your regular vitamins and herbs.

- How well your **digestive system** is functioning is also a factor. If you are not digesting well, you do not have enough enzymes or possibly hydrochloric acid to break down food properly. Taking digestive enzymes or hydrochloric acid for long periods is not a good solution, because they will take over the natural function of your body. Supplementation can be used in the short term, but you need to repair the body's natural function so it can perform its own job properly. **Digestive problems** can be addressed with the help of an acupuncturist, herbalist, or naturopath. They can give you dietary recommendations based on your unique set of health problems and constitution, and prescribe herbs to re-balance your systems.

- It is a common mis-conception that raw foods and whole grains are the healthiest way to eat. It is actually better to **cook your food** (not overcook!) in order to start the chemical breakdown process, so your digestive system doesn't have to work as hard. If you are having trouble digesting, white rice and bread are easier to digest than whole grains. Soups are nutritious and easy to digest.

- **Fasting** is hard on the digestive system. If you want to do a cleanse, use herbs and psyllium, but don't stop eating.

- Most people should not be strict vegetarians. At the very least you should eat organic eggs for a **high-quality protein** source. Most vegetarians are not very good about combining foods, and even if they are, most still seem to feel better when they add high-quality animal protein back into their diet. Plant sources contain mainly the pyridoxol form of B-6, but animal sources contain both the pyridoxal and pyridoxamine forms of B-6, and are less susceptible to the loss of the vitamin due to cooking or preserving. B-12 is *only* found in animal proteins, including dairy products. Brewer's yeast does not contain B-12, unless the yeast is grown on a special B-12-containing substrate.

- If you have **chronic diarrhea**, you will not retain food long enough in the intestines to absorb nutrients. You will need to identify and eliminate the source of diarrhea. Acupuncture, herbs, and dietary changes can often successfully address this problem.

- Excess **caffeine** increases muscle tension and trigger point irritability, leading to increased pain. Dr.'s Travell and Simons state that "... caffeine has long been known to cause a persistent contracture, or caffeine rigor, of muscle fibers. This rigor is due to enhancement by caffeine of the release of calcium from the sarcoplasmic reticulum and to interference with the rebinding of calcium ions by the sarcoplasmic reticulum." They found that caffeine in excess of 150 mg daily (more than two eight-ounce cups of regular coffee) would lead to caffeine rigor. Based on my clinical experience, some people can't even consume 150 mg without aggravating their pain. In counting your daily intake, be sure to count any caffeine in the drugs you are taking, and remember that espresso and similar drinks will have far greater amounts of caffeine. There are websites that list caffeine amounts for foods and beverages.

- **Alcohol** aggravates trigger points by decreasing serum and tissue folate levels. It increases the body's need for vitamin C, while decreasing the body's ability to absorb it. **Tobacco** also increases the need for vitamin C. In Chinese Medicine, caffeine and alcohol are said to be very "qi stagnating." **Marijuana** is very stagnating also, and stays in your system for about three months after smoking it. Stagnation is one cause of pain, therefore using any of the above substances will increase your pain level.

- Eliminating foods and beverages that aggravate your condition (such as allergins, coffee, and alcohol) may not be enough, if the underlying condition that was caused by the food has not been resolved. For example, if you have been eating damp-producing foods (like dairy and peanut butter) which has led to dampness in the muscles (as in fibromyalgia), even if you stop ingesting the food or beverage you still have dampness in the muscles that must be eliminated. Plan on avoiding the necessary foods for two months minimum *in conjunction* with acupuncture and/or herbs and other supplements, in order to determine whether eliminating the food is helpful. Many people will stop ingesting a food or drink for one week, decide it hasn't made a difference, and then re-start their regular diet. Or the food or beverage is so important to them that they'd rather have pain and other medical conditions, than give the substance up. Reaching a conclusion after one week is one way to justify continuing to ingest the substance.

- **Herbs** should be taken with the advice of a qualified practitioner. I've seen many people who have injured their digestive systems by taking too many herbs, or herbs that are improper for their conditions and constitution. What may be the correct herb for a friend or a family member may not be the correct herb for you, so seek professional advice.

- Room-temperature **water** is better than cold drinks -- if you drink something cold, your stomach has to work harder to warm it up, and it taxes the digestive system. Drink about two quarts per day, or more if you have a larger body mass or sweat a lot. A general rule of thumb for kids and adults weighing more than 100 pounds is your body weight multiplied by the number of ounces (i.e., 140 lbs. = 70 ounces). Drink at least one extra quart per day if it is very hot out, and extra water during and immediately after a work-out. If you drink *too* much water, you can deplete Vitamin B-1 (thiamine). Thirst is not necessarily a good indicator of whether or not you are dehydrated. Your urine should be a light yellow, unless you have just taken a multivitamin or B-vitamin supplement.

- **Don't drink distilled water**, because you need the minerals found in non-distilled water. If you drink bottled water, make sure you know its source, and that it is not distilled. This industry is not currently regulated, so you may need to do some research on the company.

Vitamins

- **Vitamin C** reduces post-exercise soreness and corrects the capillary fragility which leads to easy bruising. (Hint: if you don't remember how you got a bruise, you are likely bruising too easily.) It is essential for collagen formation (connective tissue) and forming bones. Vitamin C is required for synthesis of the neurotransmitters norepinephrine and serotonin, is needed for your body's response to stress, is important for immune system function, and decreases the irritability of trigger points caused by infection.

Too *much* Vitamin C can lead to watery diarrhea or non-specific urethritis. However, Vitamin C helps terminate diarrhea due to food allergies. Vitamin C daily doses above 400mg are not used by the body, and 1000mg/day increases the risk of kidney stone formation, so mega-dosing with Vitamin C is not necessary nor recommended. Women taking estrogen or oral contraceptives may need 500mg/day.

Vitamin C is likely to be deficient in smokers, alcoholics, older people (the presence of Vitamin C in the tissues decreases with age), infants fed primarily on cows' milk (usually between the ages of 6-12 months), people with chronic diarrhea, psychiatric patients, and fad dieters. Initial symptoms of deficiency include weakness, lethargy, irritability, vague aching pains in the joints and muscles, easy bruising, and possibly weight loss. In severe cases of Vitamin C deficiency (scurvy), the gums become red, swollen, bleed easily, and teeth may become loose and fall out.

Do not take Vitamin C with antacids; since Vitamin C is ascorbic acid, and the purpose of an antacid is to neutralize acid, antacids will neutralize Vitamin C and make it ineffective. Food sources include citrus fruits and *fresh* juices, *raw* broccoli, *raw* Brussels sprouts, collard, kale, turnip greens, guava, *raw* sweet peppers, cabbage, and potatoes

- **Taking too many vitamins A, D, and E, and folic acid** can cause symptoms similar to deficiencies, so don't mega-dose on those supplements unless a health care provider has determined your condition warrants it.

- **Thiamine (Vitamin B-1)** is essential for normal nerve function and energy production within muscle cells. Diminished pain and temperature sensitivity and an inability to detect vibrations indicate you are low in thiamine. You may also possibly experience calf cramping at night, slight sweating, constipation, and fatigue. B-1 is needed for proper thyroid hormone levels (see the section on Organ Dysfunction and Disease below). Abuse of alcohol reduces thiamine absorption, and absorption is further reduced if liver disease is also present. The tannin in black tea, antacid use, and a magnesium deficiency can also prevent the absorption of thiamine. Thiamine can be destroyed by processing foods, and by heating them to temperatures above 212º F (100º C). Thiamine is excreted too rapidly when taking diuretics or drinking too much water. Lean pork, kidney, liver, beef, eggs, fish, beans, nuts, and some whole grain cereals (if the hull and germ are present) are good sources of thiamine.

- **Pyridoxine (Vitamin B-6)** is important for nerve function, energy metabolism, amino acid metabolism, and synthesis of neurotransmitters including norepinephrine and serotonin, which strongly influence pain perception. Deficiency of B-6 results in anemia, reduced absorption and storage of B-12, increased excretion of Vitamin C, blocked synthesis of niacin, and can lead to a hormonal imbalance. Deficiency of B-6 will manifest as symptoms of one of the other B-vitamins, since B-6 is needed in order for all the others to perform their functions. The need for B-6 increases with age and increased protein consumption. Tropical sprue and alcohol use interfere with its absorption. Use of **oral contraceptives** increases your requirement for B-6, and impairs glucose tolerance. This can lead to depression if you don't supplement with B-6, particularly if you already have a history of depression. Corticosteroid use, excessive alcohol use, pregnancy and lactation, antitubercular drugs, uremia, and hyperthyroidism also increase the need for B-6. Sources of B-6 include liver, kidney, chicken (white meat), halibut, tuna, English walnuts, soybean flour, navy beans, bananas, and avocados. There is also some amount of B-6 present in yeast, lean beef, egg yolk, and whole wheat.

- **Cobalamin (Vitamin B-12) and Folic Acid** need to be taken together to form erythrocytes (a type of red blood cell) and rapidly dividing cells such as those found in the gastrointestinal tract, and for fatty acid synthesis used in the formation of parts of certain nerve fibers. B-12 is needed for both fat and carbohydrate metabolism. A deficiency can result in **pernicious (megaloblastic) anemia**, which reduces oxygen coming to the site of the trigger point, adding to the dysfunctional cycle and increasing pain. A deficiency of B-12 may also cause symptoms such as non-specific depression, fatigue, an exaggerated startle reaction to noise or touch, and an increased susceptibility to trigger points. B-12 is only found in animal products or supplements. Several drugs may impair the absorption of B-12, as can mega-doses of Vitamin C for long periods of time.

- A **folate deficiency** (also known as **folic acid** when in the synthetic form) can cause you to be fatigued easily, sleep poorly, and feel discouraged and depressed. It can cause "restless legs," diffuse muscular pain, diarrhea, a loss of sensation in the extremities, and you may feel cold frequently, along with a slightly lower basal body temperature than the "normal" 98.6º F (37º C). Folic acid deficiency is very prevalent and can lead to **megaloblastic anemia**. In the U.S., studies have shown that at least 15% of Caucasians are deficient, while at least 30% of African-Americans and Latinos are deficient. At least half of Canadians eat less than the dietary recommendation. Part of the problem is that 50-95% of the folate content of foods may be destroyed in food processing and preparation, so even if you eat folate sources, you may not be receiving the benefit. A necessary conversion in the digestive system is inhibited by peas, beans, citrus fruits, acidic foods, and antacids, so eat these separately from your folic acid sources. The best sources of folate are leafy vegetables, yeast, organ meat, fruit, and lightly cooked vegetables such as broccoli and asparagus. You are at greatest risk for folate deficiency if you are elderly, have a bowel disorder, are pregnant or lactating, or use drugs and alcohol regularly. Certain other drugs will also deplete folate, such as anti-inflammatories (including aspirin), diuretics, estrogens (such as birth control pills), and anti-convulsants. You must also have adequate B-12 intake in order to absorb folic acid, plus only taking one of these can mask a severe deficiency in the other.

- **Vitamin D** is required for both the absorption and the utilization of calcium and phosphorus. It is necessary for growth and thyroid function, it protects against muscle weakness, and helps regulate the heartbeat. It is important for the prevention of cancer, osteoarthritis, osteoporosis, and calcium deficiency. A mild deficiency of vitamin D may manifest as a loss of appetite, a burning sensation in the mouth and throat, diarrhea, insomnia, visual problems, and weight loss. It has been estimated that close to 90% of patients with chronic musculoskeletal pain may have a vitamin D deficiency.

Vitamin D-3 is synthesized by the skin when exposed to the sun's UV rays. Unfortunately, many people don't get enough sun exposure, especially if they live at latitudes or in climates with little sun available during the winter months. Exposing your face and arms to the sun for 15 minutes three times per week will ensure that your body synthesizes an adequate amount of vitamin D. Because the amount of exposure needed varies from person to person and also depends on geographical location, you will need to do some personal research and perhaps consult with a dermatologist to determine the proper amount for you. Food sources of vitamin D include salmon, halibut, sardines, tuna, and eggs. Other sources include dairy products, dandelion greens, liver, oatmeal, and sweet potatoes. If you take supplements, look for the D-3 form, or fish oil capsules.

Minerals

Inadequate salt, calcium/magnesium, or potassium can lead to **muscle cramping**.

- Do not entirely eliminate **salt** from your diet, especially if you sweat. You do need some salt in your diet (unless you have been instructed otherwise by your health care provider for certain medical conditions), though you don't want to overdo it either.

- **Calcium, magnesium, potassium, and iron** are needed for proper muscle function. Iron is required for oxygen transport to the muscle fibers. Calcium is essential for releasing acetylcholine at the nerve terminal, and both calcium and magnesium are needed for the contracting mechanism of the muscle fiber. Potassium is needed to get the muscle fiber quickly ready for its next contraction. Deficiency of these minerals increases the irritability of trigger points. Calcium, magnesium, and potassium should be taken together, because an increase in one can deplete the others. Also needed for good health but not as important for muscle function are zinc, iodine, copper, manganese, chromium, selenium, and molybdenum.

  It is especially important to take **calcium** for at least a few years prior to menopause to help prevent osteoporosis. Vitamin D is needed for calcium uptake. Food sources of calcium include dairy (though this is not recommended for people with damp conditions, such as fibromyalgia), salmon, sardines, seafood, green leafy vegetables, almonds, asparagus, blackstrap molasses, brewer's yeast, broccoli, cabbage, carob, collards, dandelion greens, figs, filberts, kale, kelp, mustard greens, oats, parsley, prunes, sesame seeds, tofu, turnip greens, and whey.

- Do not take Tums or other **antacids** as a source of **calcium**. Stomach acid is needed for the uptake of calcium, but an antacid neutralizes stomach acid. So even if there is calcium present, it cannot be used. If you must take an antacid, take it several hours apart from your calcium/magnesium supplement so you will maximize your mineral uptake. **Calcium channel blockers** prescribed for high blood pressure inhibit the uptake of calcium into the sarcoplasmic reticulum of vascular smooth muscles and cardiac muscles. Since this is likely also true for skeletal muscles, calcium channel blockers would also make trigger points worse, and more difficult to treat. See your health care provider to find out if you can switch to a different medication. Consider treating the underlying causes of hypertension with acupuncture, diet changes, exercise, or whatever is appropriate to your particular set of circumstances.

- **Magnesium deficiency** is less likely to occur as a result of an inadequate dietary intake in a healthy diet as it is to malabsorption, malnutrition, kidney disease, or fluid and electrolyte loss. Magnesium is depleted after strenuous physical exercise, but proper amounts of exercise coupled with an adequate intake of magnesium improves the efficiency of cellular metabolism and improves cardio-respiratory performance. Consumption of alcohol, the use of diuretics, chronic diarrhea, consumption of fluoride, and high amounts of zinc and Vitamin D increase the body's need for magnesium.

  Magnesium is found in most foods, especially dairy products (though this is not recommended for people with damp conditions, such as fibromyalgia), fish, meat, seafood, apples, apricots, avocados, bananas, blackstrap molasses, brewer's yeast, brown rice, figs, garlic, kelp, lima beans, millet, nuts, peaches, black-eyes peas, salmon, sesame seeds, tofu, green leafy vegetable, wheat, and whole grains.

- A diet high in fats, refined sugars, and too much salt causes **potassium deficiency**, as does the use of laxatives and some diuretics. Diarrhea will also deplete potassium. If you suffer from urinary frequency, particularly if your urine is clear rather than light yellow, try taking potassium. Frequent urination causes potassium deficiency, and potassium deficiency may cause frequent urination, and a cycle of depletion ensues. Food sources of potassium include fruit (especially bananas and citrus fruits), potatoes, green leafy vegetables, wheat germ, beans, lentils, nuts, dates, and prunes.

- **Iron deficiency** can lead to **anemia**, and is usually caused by excessive blood loss from a heavy menses, hemorrhoids, intestinal bleeding, donating blood too often, or ulcers. Iron deficiency can also be caused by a long-term illness, prolonged use of antacids, poor digestion, excess coffee or black tea consumption, or the chronic use of NSAID's (non-steroidal anti-inflammatory drugs, such as ibuprofen). Calcium in milk, cheese, or as a supplement can impair absorption of iron, therefore you should take your calcium supplement separately. Do not take an iron supplement if you have an infection or cancer. The body stores it in order to withhold it from bacteria, and in the case of cancer, it may suppress the cancer-killing function of certain cells.

  Early symptoms of iron deficiency include impaired work performance, fatigue, reduced endurance, and an inability to stay warm when exposed to a moderately cold environment. 9-11% of menstruating females in the U.S. are iron deficient, and the world-wide prevalence is about 15%. Iron is best absorbed with Vitamin C. Generally food sources are adequate for improving iron levels for most people. Good sources of iron include eggs, fish, liver, meat, poultry, green leafy vegetables, whole grains, almonds, avocados, beets, blackstrap molasses, brewer's yeast, dates, egg yolks, kelp, kidney and lima beans, lentils, millet, parsley, peaches, pears, dried prunes, pumpkin, raisins, rice and wheat bran, sesame seeds, and soybeans.

One of my favorite books is "*Prescription for Nutritional Healing*" by James F. Balch, M.D., and Phyllis A. Balch, C.N.C.. It has a comprehensive list of vitamins, minerals, amino acids, antioxidants, and enzymes, and food sources for each. It has sections on common disorders listing supplements needed to treat each condition, and helpful hints.

Hormonal Changes

Women are more likely than men to develop trigger points. I have noticed this is particularly true in **menopausal** women. Some teenagers (of both sexes) going through **puberty** also seem to have a tendency to develop trigger points, leading me to believe there is a connection between hormonal changes and one potential cause of trigger points.

Organ Dysfunction and Disease

Thyroid

Both **thyroid inadequacy** (also known as hypometabolism or subclinical hypothyroidism) and **hypothyroidism** will cause and perpetuate trigger points. Hypothyroid patients may experience early morning stiffness, and pain and weakness of the shoulder girdle. Both thyroid inadequacy and hypothyroidism will produce symptoms of cold (and sometimes heat) intolerance, cold hands and feet, muscle aches and pains especially with cold rainy weather, constipation, menstrual problems, weight gain, dry skin, and fatigue and lethargy. Muscles feel rather hard to the touch, and even if a patient is on a thyroid supplement, I've noticed they are still somewhat prone to trigger points, since it is hard to fine-tune the medication exactly to the amount your body would produce if you still had a healthy thyroid organ. Some studies report the prevalence of subclinical hypothyroidism to be as high as 17% in women and 7% in men. Occasionally patients with inadequate metabolism may be thin, nervous, and hyperactive, which may result in a health care provider failing to consider subclinical hypothyroidism.

Patients with low thyroid function may be **low in thiamine (Vitamin B-1)**. Before starting on thyroid medication, try supplementing with thiamine to see if that corrects your thyroid hormone levels. If you are already on thyroid medication and you start taking B-1, you may start exhibiting symptoms of *hyper*thyroidism, and your medication dosage needs to be adjusted. If you are low in B-1 at the time of starting thyroid medication, you may develop symptoms of acute thiamine deficiency, which may be misinterpreted as an intolerance to the medication. After the B-1 deficiency is corrected, you will likely tolerate the medication. You will need to supplement with B-1 prior to and during thyroid hormone therapy to avoid a deficiency. Total body potassium is low in hypothyroidism, and high in hyperthyroidism, so you may need to adjust your potassium intake also.

Smoking impairs the action of thyroid hormone and will make any related symptoms worse. Several pharmaceutical drugs can also affect thyroid hormone levels, such as lithium, anti-convulsants, those that contain iodine, and glucocorticoid steroids, so check with your pharmacist if you have been diagnosed with hypothyroidism and are taking another medication.

A simple **home test** to check your thyroid function is to place a thermometer in your armpit for 10 minutes upon waking but before getting out of bed. Normal underarm temperature for men and post-menopausal women is 98º F (36.7º C). If you are still menstruating your temperature should be around 97.5º F (36.4º C) prior to ovulation, and 98.5º F (36.9º C) following ovulation. If your temperature is lower than this, you will want to check with your health care provider. Often health care providers will only initially test the TSH level, which may still be normal if you have hypometabolism rather than hypothyroidism. A radioimmunoassay measures T3 and T4 levels, and gives a more complete picture of the thyroid function.

If you are suffering from depression, be sure to insist that your thyroid levels are tested before starting on anti-depressant medication. I've had more than one patient (especially men) where hypothyroidism was discovered only after they had been medicated for some time.

Hypoglycemia

Both **postprandial (reactive) and fasting hypoglycemia** cause and perpetuate trigger points, and make trigger points more difficult to treat. Symptoms of both are sweating, trembling and shakiness, increased heart rate, and anxiety. Activation of trigger points in the *sternocleidomastoid* muscle by a hypoglycemic reaction may lead to dizziness and headaches. If allowed to progress, symptoms can include visual disturbances, restlessness, and impaired speech and thinking. Missing or delaying a meal does not cause hypoglycemia in a healthy person. A hypoglycemic reaction to a delayed meal usually indicates a problem with the liver, adrenal glands, or pituitary gland. Postprandial hypoglycemia usually occurs two to three hours after eating a meal rich in carbohydrates, and is most like to occur when you are under high stress.

Causes will need to be identified and addressed, if possible. Symptoms will be relieved by eating smaller, more frequent meals with fewer carbohydrates, more protein, and some fat. Avoid all caffeine, alcohol, and tobacco (even second-hand smoke). If you are waking with headaches or pain or having trouble sleeping, try eating a small snack or drink a little juice before bedtime to see if it relieves your symptoms; it usually helps. Acupuncture is quite successful in stabilizing blood sugar.

Gout

Gout will aggravate trigger points and make them difficult to treat. Doctors Travell and Simons recommend keeping the gout under control and taking Vitamin C, and then subsequent treatment of trigger points will be more effective.

Sleep Problems

Pain can interrupt sleep, and interrupted sleep can perpetuate trigger points. It is useful to know whether your sleep was interrupted before your pain started, or whether your sleep was sound and restful. If your sleep was poor prior to the pain, then there is another underlying factor which needs to be addressed to help solve the problem.

Be sure you are not sleeping poorly due to being **too warm or too cold**. If you have

problems falling asleep, try improving your nutrition and your water intake first. Take a calcium/magnesium supplement before bedtime. If you are **waking easily due to noise**, try Mack's™ soft silicon earplugs (my favorite), and try breathing deeply until you fall back to sleep. If you can't stop thinking, you sleep lightly and wake frequently, you wake early and can't fall back to sleep, are menopausal, and/or have vivid and disturbing dreams, try acupuncture and Chinese herbs.

Even if you only drink **caffeine** in the morning, it still disturbs your nighttime sleep pattern, as does **alcohol**. If you choose to give up caffeine, it will take about two weeks before your energy starts to even out and you don't feel like you have to use it to get going in the morning. **Computer use in the evening** stimulates the brain and makes it hard to fall asleep and sleep restfully. If **urinary frequency** is disturbing your sleep, try acupuncture and herbs, and increasing your potassium intake.

Consider whether your **adrenal glands** could be excreting too much cortisol (the "stress hormone"). If you are continually stressed, or if you are pushing yourself too hard and push through fatigue instead of resting or taking a nap, you will excrete more cortisol and have more difficulty sleeping at night. A Naturopathic doctor can administer a saliva test for adrenal function.

Make sure you are not being exposed to **allergens** at night. Get inexpensive soft plastic covers for your pillows and mattress, since many people are allergic to mites, and they live in your bedding. If you have a down comforter or pillow, you may be allergic to the feathers, even if you are not exhibiting classic allergic symptoms, such as sneezing and itchy eyes.

Beds that are too soft can cause a lot of muscular problems, and you may not know it is too soft. Patients usually insist their mattress is firm enough, but when queried further, will admit that sleeping on a mat on the floor gives them relief when the pain is particularly bad. If this is the case, your mattress is not firm enough, no matter how much money you spent on it or how well it worked for someone else. Different people have needs for different kinds of mattresses. An all-cotton futon is very firm, and may be best for some people. The "Sleep Number" bed allows you to change the firmness and some models have an option to control firmness separately for each side of the bed. A lot of people like memory foam beds, but I personally find them too soft. Try putting some camp mats on the floor and sleeping on them for a week. If you feel better, it is time for a new, firmer mattress. Mattresses really only last about five to seven years, and should then be replaced. Some furniture stores will let you try a mattress out for a time period before making a final decision. Be sure you have a **pillow** that keeps your head in line with your spine -- not too high or too low. Sleeping on the couch should definitely be avoided.

If pain disturbs you at night, I sometimes suggest to patients that they keep their self-help ball collection by their bed so that if they wake they can work on their trigger points, and hopefully fall back to sleep once the pain is reduced. The danger in this is that *you have to be sure you don't fall asleep on the ball*! It will cut off the circulation for too long, and make the trigger points worse. It is an easy thing to do when you are fatigued and in pain, and suddenly the pain is reduced or gone, so don't use the ball in bed unless you are sure you will not fall asleep on it.

Spinal Mis-alignments and Other Problems

Vertebrae may be out-of-alignment, and need to be adjusted by a chiropractor or osteopathic physician, or mobilized by a physical therapist. Usually there is also a muscular component that caused the mis-alignment to begin with, so a combined approach of skeletal mobilization and massage or acupuncture is probably necessary for lasting relief. A chiropractor or osteopathic physician will likely take x-rays at the initial visit to evaluate your spine. If you have already had x-rays taken, bring them with you to the visit so you can avoid duplicating x-rays.

Herniated and bulging disks may be very successfully treated with acupuncture (especially Plum Blossom technique), but if you don't get some relief fairly quickly, you may want to consider surgery if you have insurance. Spinal surgery has gotten so sophisticated that many surgeries are fairly minor procedures that have you back on your feet the next day. If you have **stenosis** (a narrowing of the central spinal cord canal or the holes the nerves come out of) acupuncture will help with pain, but not the stenosis, so surgery is probably the best option. With any surgery there is a certain amount of risk, so be sure to discuss this with your operating physician, and make sure you understand the procedure. If you are still unsure, get a second opinion from another surgeon. Disc problems and stenosis need to be confirmed with an MRI.

Bone spurs and narrowed disc spaces can cause pain. But in a random sample of the population you will find many people with bone spurs and narrowed disc spaces with no pain, and many people with pain and no bone spurs or narrowed disc spaces, so don't assume these are causing your problems, even if a health care provider has made this assumption.

I always start with the assumption that trigger points are at least part of the problem, if not all of the problem, and treat accordingly. If a patient doesn't receive some relief fairly quickly, then I know there may be something else going on and I refer them to someone who can evaluate them with an x-ray or MRI.

If you have had surgery and your pain continues, trigger points are the likely culprit, and need to be treated for lasting relief. If you still do not get relief, there is a possibility the pain is due to scar tissue from the surgery compressing a nerve root, so you will need to check with your health care provider.

Laboratory Tests

Laboratory tests may be necessary to help diagnose some of the systemic perpetuating factors. With blood chemistry profiles, an elevated erythrocyte sedimentation rate (**SED Rate**) may indicate a chronic bacterial infection, polymyositis, polymyalgia rheumatica, rheumatoid arthritis, or cancer. A decreased **erythrocyte count** and/or **low hemoglobin** points to anemia. A mean corpuscular volume (**MCV**) of over 92fl indicates the likelihood of a folate or B-12 deficiency. **Eosinophilia** may indicate an allergy or intestinal parasitic infection. An increase in **monocytes** can indicate low thyroid function, infectious mononucleosis, or an acute viral infection. Increased serum **cholesterol** can be caused by a problem with low thyroid function, and a low serum cholesterol can indicate folate deficiency. High **uric acid** levels indicate hyperuricemia and possibly gout.

Iron deficiency is detected by checking the **serum ferritin** level. A **fasting blood test** is used to diagnose hypoglycemia, and an additional **glucose tolerance test** or a 2-hour postprandial blood glucose test may be used to rule out diabetes. (Measurement of **sensory**

nerve conduction velocities can help diagnose diabetic neuropathy.) A low serum total calcium suggests a calcium deficiency, but for an accurate assessment of the available calcium, a **serum ionized calcium** test needs to be performed. **Potassium** levels can be checked with a serum potassium test.

Blood tests can determine **serum levels of Vitamins B-1, B-6, B-12, folic acid, and Vitamins C and D.** Any values in the lower 25% of the normal range or below would indicate that supplementation would be helpful in the treatment of trigger points. Remember that even if serum levels of vitamins and minerals are normal, you may still wish to use supplements since tissue supplies will drop before the body allows serum levels in the blood to drop.

See the above section on Nutritional Problems for comments on the digestive system and vitamin and mineral sources. See the above section on Organ Dysfunction and Disease for a discussion of thyroid function tests. A hair analysis can detect high levels of toxic metals exposure and deficiencies in minerals. A naturopathic doctor can perform **blood tests for food allergies**. Stool samples will reveal if **parasites** are a problem.

APPENDIX B

What Are Trigger Points?

Muscle Anatomy & Physiology

Muscles consist of many muscle cells, or *fibers* bundled together by connective tissue. Each fiber contains numerous *myofibrils*, and most skeletal muscles contain approximately one thousand to two thousand myofibrils. Each myofibril consists of a chain of *sarcomeres* connected end-to-end. Muscular contractions take place in the sarcomere.

A *muscle spindle* is a sensory receptor found within the belly of a muscle. Muscle spindles are concentrated where a nerve enters a muscle, and around nerves inside the muscles. Each spindle is composed of three to twelve *intrafusal muscle fibers*, which detect changes in the length of a muscle. As the body's position changes, information is conveyed to the central nervous system via sensory neurons, and is processed in the brain. As needed, the *motor end plate* (a type of nerve ending) releases *acetylcholine*, a neurotransmitter that tells the *sarcoplasmic reticulum* (part of each cell) to release ionized calcium. The *extrafusal muscle fibers* then contract. When contraction of the muscle fibers are no longer needed, the nerve ending stops releasing acetylcholine and the calcium pump within the sarcoplasmic reticulum re-uptakes calcium.

Trigger Point Physiology: Contractions and Inflammation

One of the current theories about the mechanism responsible for the formation of trigger points is the "Integrated Trigger Point Hypothesis." If a trauma occurs or there is a large increase in the motor end plate's release of acetylcholine, an excessive amount of calcium can be released by the sarcoplasmic reticulum. This causes a maximal contracture of a segment of muscle, leading to a maximal demand for energy and impairment of local circulation. If circulation is impaired, the calcium pump doesn't get the fuel and oxygen it needs to pump calcium back into the sarcoplasmic reticulum, so the muscle fiber stays contracted. Sensitizing substances are released, causing pain and stimulation of the autonomic nervous system, resulting in a positive feedback system with the motor nerve terminal releasing excessive acetylcholine…and so the sarcomere stays contracted.

Another current theory is the "Muscle Spindle" hypothesis, which proposes that the main cause of a trigger point is an inflamed muscle spindle (Partanen, Ojala, and Arokoski, 2010). Pain receptors activate skeletofusimotor units during sustained overload of muscles via a spinal reflex pathway which connect to the muscle spindles. As pain continues, sustained contraction and fatigue drive the skeletofusimotor units to exhaustion, and cause rigor (silent spasm) of the extrafusal muscle fibers, forming the "taut band" we feel as trigger points. Because the muscle spindle itself has a poor blood supply, the contraction and inflammatory metabolites released will be concentrated inside the spindle and lead to sustained inflammation.

A ground-breaking 2008 study (Shah et al.) was able to measure eleven elevated biochemicals in and surrounding active trigger points, including inflammatory mediators, neuropeptides, catecholamines, and cytokines (primarily sensitizing substances and immune system biochemicals). In addition, the pH of the samples was strongly acidic compared to other areas of the body. A 1996 study by Issbener, Reeh, and Steen found that a localized acidic pH lowers the pain threshold sensitivity level of sensory receptors (part of the nervous system), even without acute damage to the muscle. This means the more acidic your pH level in a given area, the more easily you will experience pain compared to someone else. Further studies are needed to discover whether body-wide elevations in pH acidity and the substances mentioned above predispose people to develop trigger points.

More studies are needed to determine the exact mechanisms of trigger point formation and physiology.

Central Sensitization, Trigger Points, and Chronic Pain

The *autonomic nervous system* controls the release of acetylcholine, along with involuntary functions of blood vessels and glands. Anxiety and nervous tension increase autonomic nervous system activity, which commonly aggravates trigger points and their associated symptoms.

The *central nervous system* includes the brain and spinal cord, and its function is to integrate and coordinate all activities and responses of the body. The purpose of the *acute* stress responses of our bodies is to protect us by telling us to pull away from a hot stove burner, flee from a dangerous situation, or rest an injured body part due to pain. But when emotional or physical stress is prolonged, even just for days, there is a maladaptive response: damage to the central nervous system, particularly to the sympathetic nervous system and the hypothalamus-pituitary-adrenal (HPA) systems. This is called *central nervous system sensitization.*

Pain causes certain types of nerve receptors in muscles to relay information to *neurons* located within part of the gray matter of the spinal cord and the brain stem. Pain is amplified there and then is relayed to other muscles, thereby expanding the region of pain beyond the initially affected area. Persistent pain leads to long-term or possibly permanent changes in these neurons, which affect adjacent neurons through *neurotransmitters.*

Various substances are released: *histamine* (a compound that causes dilation and permeability of blood vessels), *serotonin* (a neurotransmitter that constricts blood vessels), *bradykinin* (a hormone that dilates peripheral blood vessels and increases small blood vessel permeability), and *substance P* (a compound involved in the regulation of the pain threshold). These substances stimulate the nervous system to release even more acetylcholine locally, adding to the perpetuation of trigger points.

Central sensitization may cause the part of the nervous system that would normally counteract pain to malfunction and fail to do its job. As a result, pain can both be more easily triggered by lower levels of physical and emotional stressors, and also be more intense and last longer. Prolonged pain caused by central nervous system sensitization can lead to emotional and physical stress. Conversely, prolonged exposure to both emotional and physical stressors can lead to central nervous system sensitization and subsequently cause pain. Just the central nervous system maladaptive changes alone can be self-perpetuating and cause pain, even without the presence of either the original or any additional stressors, creating a vicious cycle of pain and trigger point formation.

Once the central nervous system is involved, because of central sensitization, even if the original perpetuating factor causing trigger points are resolved, trigger points can continue being formed and reactivated. So the longer pain goes untreated, the greater the number of neurons that get involved and the more muscles they affect, causing pain in new areas, in turn causing more neurons to get involved…the bigger the problem becomes, leading to the likelihood that pain will become chronic. The problem gets more complex, more painful, more debilitating, more frustrating, and more time-consuming and expensive to treat. The longer you wait, the less likely you are to get complete relief, and the more likely it is that your trigger points will be reactivated chronically and periodically. The sooner pain is treated, including addressing the initiating stressors and perpetuating factors, the less likely it will become a permanent problem with widespread muscle involvement and central nervous system changes.

How Will You Know if You Have Trigger Points?

The two most important characteristics of trigger points that you will notice are tender knots or tight bands in the muscles, and referred pain. You may also notice weakness, lack of range-of-motion, or other symptoms you would not normally associate with muscular problems.

Tenderness, "Knots," and Tight Bands in the Muscle

When pressed, trigger points are usually very tender. This is because the sustained contraction of the myofibril leads to the release of sensitizing neurotransmitters via a cascade effect: the sustained contraction elevates metabolites such as potassium ions and lactic acid, which leads to the elevated levels of inflammatory agents such as bradykinin and histamine, which activates pain nerve fibers, which leads to the excretion of pain transmitters, such as substance P.

Pain intensity levels can vary depending on the amount of stress placed on the muscles. The intensity of pain can also vary in response to flare-ups of any of the perpetuating factors addressed in Appendix A, and the presence of central sensitization (see above). The areas at the ends of the muscle fibers also become tender, either at the bone or where the muscle attaches to a tendon.

Healthy muscles usually do not contain knots or tight bands, are not tender to pressure, and, when not in use, feel soft and pliable to the touch, not like the hard and dense muscles found in people with chronic pain. People often tell me their muscles feel hard and dense because they work out and do strengthening exercises, but healthy muscles feel soft and pliable when not being used, even if you work out. Muscles with trigger points may also be relaxed, so don't assume you do not have trigger points just because the muscle is *not* hard and dense.

Referred Pain

Trigger points may refer pain both in the area in which the trigger point is located, and/or to other areas of the body. These are called *referral patterns*. About half of commonly found trigger points are not located within their area of referred pain. The most common referral patterns have been well documented and diagramed, and are found in the muscle chapters in section III of this book.

Unless you know where to search for trigger points, and you only work on the areas where you feel pain, you probably won't get relief. For example, trigger points in the iliopsoas muscle (deep in your abdomen) can cause pain in your lumbar area. If you don't check the iliopsoas muscle for trigger points, and only work on the quadratus lumborum muscle in the lumbar area, you will not get relief.

There are approximately four hundred muscles in the human body, but a few muscles may or may not be present in some people. Any muscle can develop trigger points, potentially causing referred pain and other symptoms. There are also individual variations in fiber or tendon arrangement, so trigger points may be located in different places for different people.

Weakness and Muscle Fatigue

Trigger points can cause weakness and loss of coordination, along with an inability to use the muscle. Many people take this as a sign that they need to strengthen the weak muscles, but you can't condition (strengthen) a muscle that contains trigger points -- these muscle fibers are not available for use because they are already contracted. If trigger points aren't inactivated first, strengthening (*conditioning*) exercises will likely encourage the surrounding muscles to do the work instead of the muscle containing the trigger point, further weakening and deconditioning the muscle containing trigger points.

Muscles containing trigger points are fatigued more easily and don't return to a relaxed state as quickly when you stop using the muscle. Trigger points may cause other muscles to tighten up and become weak and fatigued in the areas where you experience the referred pain, and also cause a generalized tightening of an area as a response to pain.

Other Symptoms

Trigger points can cause symptoms that most people would not normally associate with muscular problems. For example, trigger points in the abdominal muscles can cause urinary frequency and bladder spasms, bed-wetting, chronic diarrhea, frequent belching and gas, nausea, loss of appetite, heartburn, food intolerance, painful menses, projectile vomiting, testicular pain, and pain that feels like it is in an organ, in addition to causing referred pain in the abdominal, mid-back, and lumbar areas.

Trigger points may also cause stiff joints, generalized weakness or fatigue, twitching, trembling, and areas of numbness or other odd sensations. It probably wouldn't occur to you (or your health care provider) that these symptoms could be caused by a trigger point in a muscle.

Sensitization of the Opposite Side of the Body

For any long-term pain, it's not unusual for both sides of the body to eventually be affected; for example, if the right lumbar area is painful, there may be tender points in the left lumbar area. Often the opposite side is actually *more* tender with pressure. This is because whatever is affecting one side is likely affecting the other: poor body mechanics, poor footwear, overuse injuries, chronic degenerative or inflammatory conditions, chronic disease, or central sensitization. For that reason, I almost always treat both sides on patients, and I recommend that you do self-treatments on both sides. You may find that you have trigger points only on one side for any given muscle, but always check both sides before making that assumption.

Active Trigger Points vs. Latent Trigger Points

If a trigger point is *active*, it will refer pain or other sensations and limit range of motion. If a trigger point is *latent*, it may cause a decreased range of motion and weakness, but not pain. The more frequent and intense your pain, the greater the number of active trigger points you likely have.

Trigger points that start with some impact to the muscle, such as an injury, are usually active initially. Poor posture or poor body mechanics, repetitive use, a nerve root irritation, or any of the other perpetuating factors addressed in Appendix A can also form active trigger points. Latent trigger points can develop gradually without being active first, and you don't even know they are there. Most people have at least some latent trigger points, which can easily be converted to active trigger points.

Active trigger points may at some point stop referring pain and become latent. However, these latent trigger points can easily become active again, which may lead you to believe you're experiencing a new problem when in fact an old problem—perhaps even something you've forgotten about—is being reaggravated. Any of the perpetuating factors discussed in Appendix A can activate previously latent trigger points and make you more prone to developing new trigger points initiated by impacts to muscles.

What Initiates and Perpetuates Trigger Points?

Trigger points may form after a sudden trauma or injury, or they may develop gradually. Common initiating and perpetuating factors are mechanical stresses, injuries, nutritional problems, emotional factors, sleep problems, acute or chronic infections, organ dysfunction and disease, and other medical conditions.

You will have more control over some perpetuating factors than others. Addressing any pertinent perpetuating factors is so important that you may obtain either a great amount or complete relief from pain without any additional treatment. If you don't eliminate perpetuating factors to the extent possible, you may not get more than temporary relief from self-help pressure techniques or practitioners' treatments. Hopefully, you will learn enough about the perpetuating factors in Appendix A that at least if you choose not to resolve them, you are making an informed choice about whether the relief of pain is more important to you than continuing to do things that make you feel worse.

You cannot realistically make all of the changes in the muscle chapters and Appendix A all at once, but make a list of the perpetuating factors that might apply to you. Prioritize and work on resolving those you think might be most important.

Other Books by the Author

Pain Relief with Trigger Point Self Help, DeLaune, Valerie LAc

Flashdrive format (2004, revised 2012, 2017). A multimedia book-on-Flashdrive for pain relief, appropriate for both practitioners and the lay public. It contains information on the causes and locations of trigger points for the entire body, along with hundreds of color photos with overlays of common pain referral patterns, and 144 video clips of self-help techniques for applying pressure to trigger points and performing stretches. A search feature allows you to search for your related medical conditions. Because the book navigates in your web browser, it is easy to locate the source of your pain, and move from one relevant chapter to the next.

It contains introductory chapters on the physiology and characteristics of trigger points, and a comprehensive chapter on all of the perpetuating factors that can cause and keep trigger points activated, along with solutions. Perpetuating factors include poor ergonomics and poorly-designed furniture, clothing problems, inadequate nutrition, inadequate water, improper diet, injuries, spinal and skeletal factors, sleep problems, emotional factors, allergies, hormonal imbalances, organ dysfunction or disease, and acute or chronic viral, bacterial, or parasitic infections. For more information on how to purchase this book, and for additional resources, go to http://triggerpointrelief.com/

Other Titles by Valerie DeLaune, LAc

Trigger Point Therapy Workbook for Upper Back and Neck Pain (2nd ed., 2013) Anchorage: Institute of Trigger Point Studies (e-pub, Print-on-Demand)

Trigger Point Therapy Workbook for Shoulder Pain including Frozen Shoulder (2nd ed., 2013) Anchorage: Institute of Trigger Point Studies (e-pub, Print-on-Demand)

Trigger Point Therapy Workbook for Lower Back and Gluteal Pain (2nd ed., 2013) Anchorage: Institute of Trigger Point Studies (e-pub, Print-on-Demand)

Trigger Point Therapy Workbook for Chest and Abdominal Pain (2013) Anchorage: Institute of Trigger Point Studies (e-pub)

Trigger Point Therapy Workbook for Headaches & Migraines including TMJ Pain (2013) Anchorage: Institute of Trigger Point Studies (e-pub)

Trigger Point Therapy Workbook for Lower Arm Pain including Elbow, Wrist, Hand & Finger Pain (2013) Anchorage: Institute of Trigger Point Studies (e-pub)

Trigger Point Therapy Workbook for Knee, Leg, Ankle, and Foot Pain (2018) Anchorage: Institute of Trigger Point Studies (e-pub, Print-on-Demand)

For more information on how to purchase these books, and for additional resources, go to http://triggerpointrelief.com/

"Like" the *author* on Facebook at Facebook.com: Valerie-DeLaune

"Like" the *Institute of Trigger Point Studies* on Facebook at Facebook.com: Institute-of-Trigger-Point-Studies